KT-437-139

THE GUT MAKEOVER

4 Weeks to Nourish Your Gut, Revolutionise Your Health and Lose Weight

JEANNETTE HYDE

Nutritional Therapist BSc.

Quercus

First published in Great Britain in 2015 by
Quercus Editions Ltd

This paperback edition published in 2016 by

Quercus Editions Ltd
Carmelite House
50 Victoria Embankment
London EC4Y 0DZ

An Hachette UK company

Copyright © 2015 Jeannette Hyde

The moral right of Jeannette Hyde to be identified as the
author of this work has been asserted in accordance with the
Copyright, Designs and Patents Act, 1988.

All rights reserved. No part of this publication may be
reproduced or transmitted in any form or by any means,
electronic or mechanical, including photocopy, recording,
or any information storage and retrieval system, without
permission in writing from the publisher.

A CIP catalogue record for this book is available
from the British Library.

PB ISBN 978 1 78429 774 9
EBOOK ISBN 978 1 78429 773 2

Every effort has been made to contact copyright holders.
However, the publishers will be glad to rectify in future
editions any inadvertent omissions brought to their attention.

Quercus Editions Ltd hereby exclude all liability to the extent
permitted by law for any errors or omissions in this book and for
any loss, damage or expense (whether direct or indirect) suffered by
a third party relying on any information contained in this book.

If you have a medical condition or suspect one, consult your
GP before following The Gut Makeover. Nothing in this
book is intended to replace or override any medical advice or
treatment you may be receiving. Author and publisher accept no
responsibility for health outcomes from the methods in this book.

10 9 8 7 6 5 4 3 2 1

Typeset by e-type, Liverpool

Printed and bound in Great Britain by Clays Ltd, St Ives plc

To Dad (Ralph Hyde 1939–2015)

MORAY COUNCIL LIBRARIES & INFO.SERVICES	
20 41 68 20	
Askews & Holts	
613.25	

Contents

Part 3: Recipes and meal plans

Part 4: Eating for Life

PART ONE

The science of gut health and the Western diet

Introduction

The media have declared that there is a revolution – and that is not too strong a word – happening right now in the nutrition world. Recent discoveries from leading researchers have shown that the state of our gut is central to our weight and health. So if we want to look and feel good for the long term, we need a diet that creates a high-performance digestive system. We have entered the gut-health era of diet and nutrition, and it will be here for a long time indeed. The science is simply too persuasive to suggest otherwise.

So, back to basics. The digestive tract is huge and tightly packed within the body. Running from mouth to anus, if it were laid out straight it would be around 7–9 metres (23–30ft) long. Our intestines, especially our large intestine, contain masses of bacteria – weighing on average 1.5kg (3½lb) in each individual, and these are instrumental to our well-being.

The collection of bacteria living on and in our body has been dubbed the 'microbiome' (see page 19) and consists of about 100 trillion bacterial cells. This is actually ten times more numerous than the human cells in the body, which means we are only 10 per cent human; the rest of us is all this stuff that is living in and on us.

The highest concentration of bacteria is to be found in our gut. Having a wide diversity of these bugs in our intestines is now understood to be essential to life. In 2014 a landmark review paper on the microbiome published in the *Journal of Clinical Investigation* from New York University said: 'The composition of the microbiome and its activities are involved in most, if not all, of the biological processes that constitute human health and disease, as we proceed through our own life cycle.'

Until now our gut health has been totally underestimated, but we now know that it is essential to take care of it from cradle to old age. It amazes me that it has taken so long for the idea of gut health to have a revolution. When Hippocrates (circa 460–375 BC) said 'bad digestion is the root of all evil' he was certainly on to something all those centuries ago.

Good gut health has an important impact on many aspects of your health, some of which might not have occurred to you:

- There is a growing body of research showing that not all calories are created equal. Junk food, sugar, artificial sweeteners, alcohol and meat reared on antibiotics may change the balance of bacteria in the gut and actually make us extract more calories from them than unprocessed foods – even if the calorie counts are the same.

- The digestive system has now been dubbed 'the second brain' – with signals passing from gut to brain, not just the other way round as originally thought. This may mean an unhealthy gut playing a role in a low mood, and a healthy gut doing the same for a better mood.

- A disturbed gut lining can lead to undigested particles of food, or toxins, getting into our bloodstream, leading to irritated skin, allergy-style symptoms and a confused immune system.

- A healthy microbiome has been linked with a healthy immune system. The microbiome is in contact with a large pool of the immune system – around 70 per cent of immune cells live in the gut.

The great news is there is a lot you can do to cultivate a healthy gut. The biggest influence you can have on the state of your gut lining, and a healthy microbiome, is your diet – which *you* control.

So what does this mean for us in practice? Simply, it means that we need to adopt a diet which stimulates the flourishing of as many different and varied species of gut bugs as possible, and which makes the beneficial bugs bloom and thrive. We also need to put foods into our diet daily that we know will help us to build a strong gut lining. Both of these concepts have recently been shown to be key to controlling weight, beautiful skin, improving mood and developing a strong immune system. A good gut may also protect us from developing autoimmune disorders, which are currently at near-epidemic levels in developed countries.

This book will explain how to eat to achieve great gut health, even in your busy life. It will set you on the path to strengthening your gut lining and reseeding the bugs in your intestines to give you vibrant health and achieve a body weight that suits you.

How the makeover works

The book centres around a four-week plan that I have designed based on the latest research on the microbiome and impaired intestinal permeability (also known as leaky gut, see page 26). It is not a diet in the popular sense of the word; it is a restoration programme. It's a whole health overhaul.

For four weeks we are going to take out of your everyday diet the foods which could be irritating your gut lining or skewing the balance and impacting the diversity of that 1.5kg (3½lb) of bacteria in your intestines, and replace them with foods which will help. Think of it as a personal makeover working from the inside out; using good food to restore your bacteria, to create a knock-on impact on your weight, skin, mood and immune system.

The four-week plan pays a nod to the diets of indigenous hunter-gatherers, in South America and Africa, who have a wide range of species of bacteria in their guts supported by eating many vegetables, and supplemented with quality meats and fish, eggs, nuts and seeds, and from time to time, a little dairy. The plan involves eating a diverse array of delicious, unprocessed foods which won't leave you hungry.

Once we have built your gut up to a state of bacterial diversity and abundance on the four-week makeover, we will transition to the maintenance part of this programme, which is a gut-friendly version of the real Mediterranean diet, based on the diet from the pre-1960s in Greece. This consisted of a high intake of plants – vegetables, seasonal fruits and wild herbs – supplemented with fish, nuts and grains, extra virgin olive oil, artisan, slow-matured cheeses teeming with friendly bacteria and moderate amounts of quality meat. This Mediterranean diet can support a healthy gut. It's also an enjoyable way to eat for the long term.

By following this plan you will implement a set of habits that you can incorporate into your diet every day. Once you have a strong gut lining and a flourishing, healthy pond of beneficial bacteria, you will go forward with a set of principles to keep it that way. The recommendations in these pages are simple and implementable, so you can attain and maintain a tip-top-condition gut and enjoy good health and weight even after the four weeks are up. You may from time to time come back to the four-week plan. It isn't a roller coaster of feast and famine, self-denial and rebound hunger, it's simply a hit of the reset button.

The Gut Makeover is enjoyable and easy to follow, and its recipes accessible and filling, but if you need a little convincing to carry on with the diet, all the way through I will provide you with explanations of the ground-breaking research behind it. I will share with you the latest digestive health science, coupled with my clinical experience based on it, to help you improve your weight and general health. This is a massive area of research, expanding by the day, with the biggest advances having occurred within the past three years (1,389 research papers on 'gut microbiome' were published on the PubMed database in the first seven months of 2015, compared to 389 in 2010 and 55 in 2005). Many of the findings are discussed behind closed doors at medical conferences and in peer-reviewed scientific literature; applying it to real life is my job and my passion. I have assessed this research and designed a style of eating for one month which will help you build a strong gut lining, and reseed the bugs in your intestines for vibrant health. So, let's grab hold of this revolutionary gut science and adopt an eating pattern to improve your health today.

Buzzword bugbears

I'd like to mention my two language irritations around healthy eating: the phrase 'going on a diet' and the word 'clean'. Let's first start with 'going on a diet'. For me, this phrase spells misery, depravation and starvation. It also spells short-termism. It also in my experience, and the experience of many people I have met, often carries connotations of failure. That is why I like to talk about having a 'plan' or 'eating strategy' rather than 'being on a diet'.

The second buzzword that grates is eating 'clean'. This is the new term you see a lot on websites and spoken among evangelical communities who are doing something I do agree with – shunning processed food and eating natural, unprocessed food instead. Brilliant! But if you call that clean, does that mean when you're not eating that way you're eating dirty? And how does that make you feel – a failure? As you'll find out later in this book, I don't want you to eat processed food, as you are unlikely to reach your goals with it. While I agree with the idea behind eating 'clean' (avoiding processed foods) I have not adopted this word as I find it judgemental and confusing. So in this book, you won't see the word 'clean', but you will hear me encouraging you to choose unprocessed foods wherever possible.

The life-changing benefits

To call *The Gut Makeover* a diet – a word most people associate with slimming – would acknowledge just one small part of the benefits you are likely to see from undergoing this makeover for a month. On this plan your gut undergoes a restoration programme along with the rest of your health. You may find you experience fewer niggly ailments, too.

The people who have tried *The Gut Makeover* have seen a large number of benefits, including: increased energy, better mood and fewer mood swings, less anxiety, less bloating and tummy fat, better sleep, fewer aches and pains, disappearance of swollen ankles, reduction or disappearance of menopausal symptoms such as hot flushes, improvement in constipation, disappearance of heartburn, improvement in asthma and hay fever, disappearance of acne and mouth ulcers, and complete subsidence of food cravings – and that's all before even losing weight!

Weight loss

Benefit: Most people will lose 6–13lb (3–6kg) in the first month, but if the key principles are maintained longer term this can continue gradually in the months afterwards, with weight stabilisation going forward.

Why?: Research shows that if our microbiome has a low bacteria count and certain friendly species are not dominating we may extract more calories from our diet – whatever that may be. We may also feel hungrier. Many of us have a depleted microbiome because antibiotics have wiped out some of the beneficial bacteria and we are eating a poor diet. One course of antibiotics can leave the microbiome weaker for up to four years, leading to increased calorie extraction and appetite changes. However, rebuilding the numbers of different species of bacteria in our gut with the right food could reverse this. The microbiome can be recalibrated in days to weeks through *The Gut Makeover*.

Better mental health

Benefit: Most people experience a better mood and a reduction in mood swings, anxiety, fear, nervousness, aggressiveness, irritability, anger and depression.

Why?: The gut has been dubbed 'the second brain' and it has more than 100 million neurons embedded in its walls. We all know how our mood can impact our gut – for instance, experiencing butterflies when we are nervous. But it is now understood that hormonal and neural signals pass from the gut to the brain, which means that if the bacteria in our gut is out of balance, or the numbers of species are low, our mood and thinking may be affected. *The Gut Makeover* will put foods into your diet to help friendly gut bacteria flourish and the breadth of species rise.

Improved immune system

Benefit: People experience improvements in gut complaints and immune disorders, such as reduced bloating, heartburn, constipation, loose stools as well as less pain and symptoms connected with autoimmunity, such as rheumatoid arthritis, psoriatic arthritis and psoriasis.

Why?: Our gut bacteria send messages to our immune cells, so having a diverse range of bacterial species can support the immune system and prevent us catching every cough and cold going. Supporting our gut bacteria, and therefore our immune system, through *The Gut Makeover* can also reduce our risk of autoimmune disorders, currently at near-epidemic levels – with more than 80 known at time of writing.

Better skin

Benefit: Many find an improvement in acne, hives, eczema, rashes and rosacea.

Why?: To have beautiful skin we need to support our microbiome. A bag of healthy gut flora has been linked with healthy skin.

My gut story

For decades we've all been counting calories – in, out, in, out, shake it all about. Be honest now, how many calorie-controlled diets have you been on in your lifetime? Me? More than I care to remember! The first was in the 1980s, when I was 18. I looked in a mirror and thought (of course, mistakenly) that if I was thinner I'd look better and people might like me more. At the time I was very influenced by all the chitter-chatter among my peers about weight loss and perfectionism. So I bought a little yellow book listing calorie counts and became such an expert that I could calculate the numbers of every meal without even looking at it any more.

Over a few months I became thinner and thinner. At 170cm (5ft 7in) tall I went from a healthy 9½ stone (60kg) to about 8 stone (51kg). Then one day I woke up and suddenly had the most insatiable hunger of my life. I couldn't stop eating and started craving junk foods I had never eaten before. I remember being on the upstairs of a bus and turning my head to see a McDonald's; I immediately had to break my journey, get off and go in and have a big binge. I would buy a loaf of sliced white bread, a pot of jam and some margarine, saying to myself I'd have just one slice, but then I'd sit by the toaster preparing each one till the entire loaf was gone in one sitting.

I gained 3½ stone (22kg) and rocketed to 11½ stone (73kg) – the heaviest I have ever been before or after that time. Instead of being thin, I was now officially overweight for my height. I felt permanently depressed, my skin was a mess, I caught several colds a year and my figure was destroyed – along with any tiny piece of confidence I'd ever harboured. My thighs rubbed together painfully when I walked, and I lived in a long black sack jumper to hide my shape.

It took me another four years of misery-bingeing and crash-dieting, counting calories then giving up, and punishing exercise routines before I managed to break the cycle. That was when I finally gave up calorie counting once and for all. The main person behind this change was my mother, who kept pushing me to 'eat properly', as she put it. And you know what? I got my weight back in balance. For four months I ate three balanced meals a day, which consisted of meat, fish and a large variety of vegetables – many from my dad's garden. I also bravely went back to eating butter rather than avoiding fats, had a boiled egg for breakfast and ate live yoghurts at the same time each day. I also walked a dog every day for an hour. I never went hungry. Soon I dropped back to my 18-year-old weight of 9½ stone (60kg) that I'd been before all this misery and distress began. Why did it work, without counting calories? At the time I had no idea, but when we see what is emerging about the microbiome today I realise that it is probably what holds the answer.

I have to admit, I didn't totally learn my lesson. During a period of chronic stress and self-neglect while I was working on national newspapers, 16 years later in the early 2000s, I did put on weight – but not in the same proportions. Back then I was eating lunch at my desk, grabbing sandwiches from a trolley which would park behind me several times a day. For breakfast each day I would guzzle coffee while shoving a croissant into my mouth on a crowded station platform. After a while, in desperation, I resorted to calorie counting again. Spurred on by popular nutrition mantras of the time, I started replacing full-fat items for reduced-fat ones in the belief this would make me thinner. This was the science at that time; calories in, calories out, replace full-fat with low-fat and high-calorie foods with artificial sweeteners and you'll be thin. But it was always a short-term fix followed by rebound hunger and weight gain. I found myself struggling with my weight, skin, mood and immune system, catching every cough and cold going. When I left journalism nine years ago, I gave up dieting, and with it poor health. My motivation was a mixture of failing health and a personal crusade for the truth about food, which then drove me to study nutrition.

Since that epiphany I have discovered that it is impossible to ever know the whole truth about food – research will continue to open this field decade after decade with more and more new discoveries and breakthroughs. But often one area of research is better put into context by the next chunk of research, like putting a puzzle together.

My late mother was a big influence on me moving into nutrition. I used to be ribbed mercilessly in the 1970s at school about my rather alternative background, and I was deeply embarrassed about it at the time. My mother would stand at the school gates in Lewisham, south-east London, with her henna-dyed hair, sporting a Native American striped poncho – the stick I got for that! We ate Cranks brown bread at a time when white sliced really was the next big thing, and we always had 'live' yoghurt, though I didn't know why. Dinners were nut and lentil bakes and pick-your-own vegetables, which we drove to gather from the Kent countryside in our clapped-out, dark-green VW Beetle at various times of the year. Later, home-grown vegetables were a big part of family life. For many years I refused to eat anything home-grown because I hated being 'different'. Why couldn't we have white bread and buy food in packets like 'normal' families?

In adult life, however, when I was eating on the station platform and grabbing rubbish from the trolley, and feeling rubbish too, I knew that, although my mother hadn't had a science degree, she certainly knew a lot about the common-sense diet and how to get nutrient-dense food into her family. I now know that brown bread hasn't had the best part of the kernel with the B vitamins stripped out of it, and that we need those B vitamins for good mental health and to make energy in the body. These important B vitamins are also manufactured in the gut by our gut bacteria, and live yoghurt and lots of vegetables certainly helps that happen.

So when my health started stalling as an adult, and I started trying to work out how to be healthy, I became frustrated. I wanted to get to the truth about food, to be able to critique first-hand scientific research for myself and interpret it into practice. This led me to doing a four-year BSc course in nutritional therapy at the University of Westminster, and, after graduating in 2012, entering nutritional therapy private practice and writing on nutrition. This book is the culmination of the last nine years of my work.

One thing I've learnt on my own personal weight-management journey is that putting good eating into practice every day is something you have to keep focused on – not just the week before a holiday, or in January after Christmas. Self-care is ongoing, and if you're doing it right, you get better and better at it, adding new techniques here and using new knowledge and better tools there.

A road map of the gut

To put my ideas into context, let's have a quick tour of the digestive system. The tube that runs continuously from mouth to anus is a major highway passing through the body. It is finally beginning to be acknowledged that much of our health is dependent on this highway performing optimally. A problem near the beginning of the journey, such as the mouth or stomach, can have a big impact on the gut lining and bacteria balance further down. This becomes clearer when we see what happens when it is operating well.

The mouth

The first stage of digestion happens in the mouth itself. This is where the mechanical breakdown of food occurs, as we grind and chew it with our teeth. Digestion is also aided by the release of enzymes; these are like chemical scissors, snipping food into smaller molecules so that they can be absorbed into our bloodstream further down the line. Some of these enzymes are released in our saliva. We often start producing saliva when we smell good food, or see attractive food, which is why both cooking food and eating it slowly can help our digestion – rather than just throwing it in a microwave for a minute and eating it out of a container at our desk between responding to urgent emails.

The stomach

Once the food has been broken down by the teeth and mixed around with saliva, it goes down the chute (the oesophagus) to the stomach, which is like a stretchy balloon sitting behind our ribs. The stomach is a dynamic organ, which can stretch in size to accommodate larger quantities of food. It produces hydrochloric acid and more enzymes, which work to further break down the arriving food, spontaneously tossing the food around in a churning action so it gets really well mixed in with the acid and the enzymes – rather like a washing machine. The mashed-up food is then pumped through to the next chamber gradually. By now it's pretty sludgy.

It usually takes about four to four and a half hours for a meal to leave the stomach. When our stomach is empty, it produces a hunger hormone called ghrelin, which lets the brain know it is time to eat again. When the stomach is stretched and full, the secretion of ghrelin stops, giving us that sensation of feeling full.

The small intestine

I can never get my head around why the small intestine is called small when it is so long – on average it is 6–7 metres (20–23ft) long (or as tall as a two-storey building). When the food enters your small intestine it should now be sludge – as long as you chew properly and your digestive enzyme and acid production are working well. This sludge is now known as 'chyme'. At this point, bile and more digestive enzymes join the chyme to help break it down into smaller and smaller particles. The food takes three to six hours to pass through this tube, and this is where the big, important action of absorption happens. This is how all the fuel and nutrients get into our bloodstream. The sludge is squeezed along by automatic contractions called peristalsis; these are very important because if they slow down, for example in the days after a general anaesthetic, we can become constipated.

The sludge has quite a way to go. The texture of the inside of this long tube looks like a shag-pile carpet: each strand is dotted with microvilli, which look like the bristles on a brush and are, unsurprisingly, known as the brush border. The shag pile and brush hairs have been designed to provide an enormous surface area for ease of absorption. If all the strands of shag pile (villi) and brush border (microvilli) were stretched out flat, the small intestine would have the surface area of a tennis court.

Our shag-pile carpet gets a huge amount of traffic every day, so it can wear out quickly, but when we are healthy, cells turn over quickly and good-quality replacements are constantly being built. The inside of this tube is also covered in slimy mucus, which is produced from goblet cells. This helps protect the carpet and keep potentially pathogenic bacteria from passing through into the bloodstream. Of course, we can't see the texture and health of our inner small intestine (without a medical procedure), but if it isn't functioning right – if the shag pile and brush texture get worn down, the junctions between the shags come loose or torn, or if there is less mucus than normal – our absorption, and consequently our whole health, can be compromised.

After the enzymes and bile have all done their work and the sludge has been completely broken down to the lowest common denominator, the nutrients go through the little junctions between the blades of the brush border and shag piles into our bloodstream to fuel us and the leftovers are transferred to the large intestine.

The large intestine – and the microbiome

The large intestine or the colon is the final stop after the small intestine. This long tube is shorter and fatter than the small intestine, and is where any water is absorbed. The residues – think of vegetables with particularly hard-to-break-down strands and material – provide food for the trillions of microbes. These leftovers spend up to two days in this department before they are excreted from the body.

In science, the colon used to be a forgotten and dismissed part of the digestive system, until the microbiome came along. Of course, this pond of bacteria had always been there, it just hadn't had much recognition before. Scientists are now calling the microbiome 'the forgotten organ'. For decades, bacteria in the gut were considered benign or fairly insignificant, but between 2008 and 2012 scientists across the US participated in large-scale research, The Human Microbiome Project, to examine and identify much of this bacteria in healthy people. Bacteria runs through the whole digestive system, but the majority of it – about 1.5–2kg (3½–4½lb) per person – lives here in the colon.

So what do these microbes do?

- They ferment indigestible fibres from plants such as vegetables to release short-chain fatty acids. The short-chain fatty acid from fibre you will hear most about is called butyrate. This is a fuel needed to build the mucus which lines the gut. The mucus protects the gut lining, which is vital for a healthy immune system, mental health and good skin. So if you don't eat enough vegetables you won't have enough fuel to build a healthy mucus layer – and without enough mucus, you are more likely to develop a leaky gut (see page 26) and suffer from ill health.

- They may determine how aggressively calories are extracted from the food we eat.
- They interact with our hormones – particularly the ones that tell us we are full or hungry.
- They manufacture B vitamins, which are needed for good mental health and to make us feel energised.
- They make vitamin K, which is needed to clot our blood if we have an accident, a cut or a graze.
- They interact with our immune cells.
- They interact with our nervous system.

The microbiome

- The microbiome is now considered a whole organ in its own right.
- Officially, there are two terms: 'microbiome' and 'microbiota' – the gut microbiota being a community of microbes and the gut microbiome being the bacteria and their associated genes together – however, researchers tend to use the two terms interchangeably.
- Between 1,000 and 1,150 species of bacteria are able to live in the human gut, containing more than 3 million genes (150 times more than human genes). The bacterial genes are

thought to interact with our human genes to switch them on or silence them. It is early days in this research, but if this is found to be true, it must therefore be essential to cultivate a healthy microbiome through our diet.

- Each person harbours at least 160 species of bacteria and the make-up of bacteria is personalised like a fingerprint. The abundance and diversity of the flora is highly influenced by diet.

- What appears to be significant to weight management and health is bacterial diversity: the greater the numbers of different species living in your gut, and consequently the greater your array of bacterial genes, the better. We need to aim for a high number of bacterial species and consequently high gene count. The best way to achieve this is through a wide and varied diet which includes many vegetables.

Gut problems

So we know what the digestive system looks like when the structure is all in good working order and it is functioning fine. But what does it look like when things go wrong? Here are the main potential problems:

IBS

Irritable bowel syndrome (IBS) is a catch-all term used by the medical profession to diagnose digestive problems where the cause is unknown. Often laboratory tests, x-rays and biopsies have come back negative. 'IBS' patients often have constipation, or loose stools, or alternate between the two. There is thought to be a stress and emotional component involved and sometimes this can indeed be the main underlying factor. However, in my clinical practice, I've seen many times, that what has been labelled 'IBS' is actually impaired intestinal permeability or dysbiosis. In my experience, removing the root cause of those (poor diet or foods an individual may be intolerant to) and implementing a gut-friendly diet (*Gut Makeover* style) often leads to a vast improvement in IBS symptoms.

Dysbiosis

I've described the microbiome as a teeming pond of life, with different communities and species of bacteria living in it. When we eat a gut-friendly diet this pond will be in a happy balance. This is an eco-system of life. We want this system to be in balance, with all the friendly bacteria blooming and proliferating. When this happens, it means the friendly bacteria ('commensal bacteria') are likely to be dominant and the unfriendly bacteria ('pathogens'), the lurgies, are kept in the background. If the lurgies become dominant, this is when we can run into health problems.

When the baddies are getting the upper hand, this picture is called 'dysbiosis'. One of the first things a person may notice with dysbiosis is their abdomen might bloat, and they may experience more wind than usual. Others might find they start catching colds because their immune system is affected, or they might feel emotionally low. Dysbiosis has been linked with low mood and anxiety. It used to be thought that mood disorders were solely to do with imbalances in the brain but recent research indicates they can be connected with disharmony in the gut. It is now known that the brain picks up on dysfunction in the gut; this is believed to be via the vagus nerve, which connects the two, as well as through hormonal and neural signals. Another consequence of dysbiosis is skin complaints, such as breaking out in spots or a worsening of eczema. Dysbiosis is also thought to result in greater numbers of calories being extracted from the food we eat.

Not chewing our food properly can also lead to undigested particles of food reaching the colon, where the non-beneficial bacteria feed on the undigested food (which isn't supposed to be there) and proliferate. Also if the stomach doesn't produce as much acid as it should do, the breakdown of food is compromised and the chance of undigested food reaching the colon and causing dysbiosis is increased. An indication of low stomach acid can be heartburn (see box).

Heartburn

Heartburn is often presumed to be the result of high stomach acid, but this is not necessarily always the case. Heartburn, or acid reflux, is where acid from the stomach pops up through the sphincter (plug hole) to your oesophagus and creates a burning sensation. It can happen when stomach acid production is low and proteins stay in the stomach longer than is normal because there isn't enough acid to break them down properly. What acid is there, with the overstaying proteins, can start to cause digestive discomfort and a burning sensation in the oesophagus.

You can stimulate the production of stomach acid by chewing your food thoroughly and putting certain foods in your diet at the start of a meal – habits you'll be practising in the four-week plan (see pages 85 and 90).

Another cause of heartburn (acid reflux) can be a sensitivity to gluten, which can develop at any stage of life. If gluten really is your particular trigger for heartburn, you may see an end to the discomfort in a matter of days of going completely gluten-free (see page 00 for more on this).

Low numbers of different species

Obese individuals have been shown to have a lower number of different species living in their guts than non-obese individuals. Why are we concerned about this? Because a large diversity of different species of bacteria living in the gut has been linked with healthy weight. Eating a diet that incorporates a wide range of plants every day will create a wide diversity of different species of bacteria to flourish and call your colon home. British people eat on average just four portions of vegetables and fruit a day. In *The Gut Makeover*, we will massively increase your plant intake, to boost the diversity of your bacteria and create an abundance of friendly-gut bacteria, and consequently modulate your weight.

The connection between weight and gut bacteria is a rapidly expanding area of research, and the links with weight are alarming. Bear with me for the rest of this paragraph – it isn't exactly conversation fodder for dinner parties, but the science is extraordinary . . . For some years, scientists have known that when they insert the faeces of slim mice, which are teeming with the bacteria from the colon, into obese mice, the obese mice become slim. When they insert the faeces of the obese mice into the slim mice's guts, the slim mice become obese. This procedure is called a faecal transplant, and has been shown in humans to be more than 90 per cent effective at curing the chronic diarrhoeal infection *Clostridium difficile*, which is usually caused by overuse of antibiotics. One unexpected side effect, though, can be an impact on weight. A recent case study saw a woman of normal weight become obese after undergoing a faecal transplant from her obese daughter. Gut bacteria is clearly powerful stuff. The lady in question's *C. difficile* was cured, but her weight became out of control. Doctors have since been advised not to use obese donors for such transplants.

Old age and species diversity

Our microbiome diversity peaks in adulthood and declines as we enter old age. If you want to counteract the loss of diversity in the gut and the subsequent weakening of your immune system as you age, you need to eat a gut-supporting diet – starting with *The Gut Makeover*.

Leaky gut (impaired intestinal permeability)

For years 'leaky gut', or – to give it the correct medical term – 'impaired intestinal permeability', was considered an invention of alternative medicine. However, there is now a large body of research that explains the mechanisms behind it. The latest review paper from Germany in 2014 references 265 research papers related to the subject.

So what is leaky gut? In our tour of the digestive system I described the inside lining of the small intestine as being like a shag-pile carpet. When we're healthy (and chew our food properly) our food should break down to the lowest common denominator of particles and then go through the shag-pile carpet, through minuscule gaps called tight junctions. However, these gaps can become wider, or ripped. If this happens, undigested particles of food, or toxins, can seep through the shag pile into our bloodstream, which causes our immune system to go into a state of alarm.

The rips or gaps can occur for a number of reasons. Perhaps we haven't chewed well, or our stomach isn't producing enough stomach acid at the moment. It could be that we are stressed or drink a lot of alcohol. We may be continuing to eat foods that our body can no longer tolerate – for some this might be foods containing wheat or other grains, or particular dairy products. Then there are the foods that haven't been broken down properly – the ten pints of lager we drank last night, or our high-wheat diet of toast, pasta and pizza we've had for breakfast, lunch and dinner that can become potential irritants to the gut lining.

So let's say you had a cream cake instead of lunch and the superhighway of your digestive system isn't operating as it should. The cream will reach your small intestine with the proteins still not broken down to the lowest common denominator of single-block amino acids. Your shag pile is ripped and so proteins, and/or peptides from the cream, will pass through the rips into your bloodstream. Suddenly your immune system goes into overdrive. Proteins? You're not supposed to be here! Invader alert! Suddenly immune cells start charging into action to fight the invader that they sense is a foreign body that shouldn't be here. They get out their weapons and start attacking the unwanted visitor. This may display itself to you as violent sneezing, a worsening of asthma, or itchy skin, chronic acne or chronic inflammation of many kinds – from obesity to depression. (For more on inflammation see the box on p. 29).

A healthy microbiome has been shown to help prevent leaky gut and reverse it. By following *The Gut Makeover*, you will remove potential gut-lining irritants to give the villi and microvilli time to repair. Instead you will eat foods that will help with the restoration of the gut-lining cells and beneficial bacteria in the colon.

Dysbiosis and leaky gut have been connected with:

- Obesity
- Eczema
- Asthma
- Acne
- Depression
- Anxiety
- Insomnia
- Type 2 diabetes and insulin resistance
- Inflammatory bowel diseases such as Crohn's and ulcerative colitis
- Irritable bowel syndrome
- Autism
- Autoimmune disorders – including multiple sclerosis, coeliac disease, psoriasis, rheumatoid arthritis, type 1 diabetes
- Parkinson's disease
- Alzheimer's
- Colorectal cancer
- Oesophageal cancer
- Cardiovascular disease

  For references and further reading on these, see page 235

Food intolerances

We can develop problems digesting certain food types when we are overexposed to them, particularly if we have a genetic predisposition (e.g. coeliac disease or non-coeliac gluten sensitivity, see page 46). This can cause an array of nasty symptoms such as gas, bloating and indigestion. Food intolerances can also lead to other gut problems such as leaky gut, which can in turn lead to dysbiosis.

A common problem food group is dairy. For example, it is estimated that 80 per cent of individuals of Asian heritage have difficulties digesting the natural sugar in milk called lactose. The genes of many cultures in Europe have adapted to tolerating dairy foods over the last 10,000 years, and lactase persistence (the production of the enzyme to break down lactose beyond infancy when it is needed to digest breast milk) has become common. In many Asian and African cultures, where dairy farming was less adopted, genes have not adapted so frequently to persistently produce lactase into adulthood.

The Gut Makeover removes common triggers of digestive discomfort such as gluten and all other grains for one month. Milk products are removed for the first fortnight and put back into the diet in prescriptive amounts in the second fortnight. At the end of the month, common allergens such as gluten, and other grains are gradually reintroduced to help you identify if any particular ones are a problem for the individual you are. The aim is to find a tailormade diet that fits your particular physiology in the long term.

What is inflammation and why should I care?

Inflammation can be a protective response in the body. For example, you fall over and break your arm and it immediately balloons into a swollen, red, painful, stiff immovable trunk. Inflammatory immune cells come to take care of the mess and fight off any foreigners (such as dirt or infectious bacteria) that might have perforated the injury and chemicals called cytokines signal pain so you don't move your arm and instead allow healing to take place.

Acute inflammation can be a helpful and useful service, but if the body keeps thinking it is injured, or that foreigners may be in its territory, this can trigger long-term inflammation that's detectable in your bloodstream called 'systemic inflammation'. Your immune system could, for instance, start mounting an immune reaction every time you eat a food you might be sensitive to (such as gluten) or if undigested particles of food are entering the bloodstream because you have leaky gut. Dysbiosis can also lead to systemic inflammation. When the gut bacteria is in balance it is thought to promote anti-inflammatory signalling to the immune system.

Systemic inflammation is implicated in autoimmune disorders. When the immune system becomes confused, immune cells start to attack cells in your own body, rather than foreign ones – for instance in psoriasis, when your immune cells start attacking your own skin, or multiple sclerosis, where immune cells attack the myelin sheaths on your nerves, which prevents nerve signalling working properly.

Systemic inflammation has also been linked with heart disease, and a mounting body of evidence indicates that inflammation is more dangerous than total cholesterol levels themselves. There are plenty of doctors talking loudly about this in the mainstream and in literature right now. Pioneering cardiologist Dr Aseem Malhotra was the bravest, starting the debate in this country with his article in the *British Medical Journal* in 2013, entitled: 'Saturated fat is not the major issue'. This made the front covers of several national newspapers that day.

As nutritionists we'd been watching the research on this coming out for several years, but no cardiologist seemed brave enough to collate and shout about it publicly in the UK. In fact, 75 per cent of patients in this country who are admitted to hospital with a heart attack have completely normal total cholesterol levels. It is becoming apparent that what is much more dangerous than total cholesterol levels is if your arteries are inflamed – which means certain types of small particle-size cholesterol (as opposed to the fluffy, big type) stick to them.

Expect to hear much more about systemic inflammation in coming years. Government advice follows scientific research, not the other way around, and it can sometimes take several decades for new findings to become adopted and accepted in mainstream medicine and translated into public health advice. Especially when it involves having to admit previous advice wasn't spot on. If I was a share-buying kind of person (which I'm not) I'd be investing in extra virgin olive oil, which has been shown to be anti-inflammatory, and probiotic foods like kefir (which have also been shown to reduce inflammation) above pharmaceutical company shares any day!

The Western diet

In the last few decades we have lost many gut-supportive habits and foods. Traditional staples such as slow-cooked stews and cheap cuts of meat such as organ meats have become scarce, as have the habits of eating meat (or fish) and two veg, regularly eating greens, eating fish on Fridays, making chicken stock from leftover bones, drinking live yoghurts or fermented foods, and eating slow-produced quality breads such as sourdoughs and smelly cheeses. Instead a typical modern Western diet is based around convenience foods and packaged items.

Here are some of the food and drink items that are most commonly found in our diets:

1. **Refined carbohydrates** – such as white bread, pasta, rice and breakfast cereals. These are quickly broken down into sugar in the body.
2. **Sugar** – from white sugar in biscuits, cakes and breakfast cereals to high-fructose corn syrup in fizzy drinks. You'll even find sugar in high doses in 'healthy' muesli bars. High-sugar diets have been linked with an impoverished microbiome.
3. **Trans fats** – these fats can be found in some commercial and highly processed cakes, biscuits, muffins, etc. and in some margarines and low-fat spreads. They can also be produced

when oils are heated repeatedly to high temperatures with deep frying. They come under names such as 'partially hydrogenated' fats and can sometimes be hard to spot. When you buy a muffin without packaging on it – say, in a coffee shop – you won't necessarily see ingredients labelling 'partially hydrogenated oils' because food packed on the premises doesn't, according to The Food Standards Agency, have to be labelled as it is assumed you can ask the owner or server. Trans fats are the ones that cause most concern in connection to heart disease and brain function; the specific chemical structure of them makes it difficult for the body to deal with them. Trans fats have been shown to raise inflammation markers, and, as mentioned on page 29, systemic inflammation has now been linked with heart disease and depression. However, although processed oils in trans fats are the most dangerous, too much fat in the diet may not be compatible with a healthy microbiome. High-fat diets have been linked with lower bacterial species in the gut, and for optimum health we want a high bacterial count. This means we should choose our fats carefully and combine them with plants for a healthy microbiome. We should look for quality and purity, selecting natural fats such as extra virgin olive oil, butter and coconut oil, as opposed to chemically manufactured fats such as those whose molecular structure changes to a trans fat during repeated deep frying or chemical manufacture.

4. **Artificial sweeteners** – from aspartame to saccharin and sucralose. We think we are only consuming them when we have diet colas and fizzy drinks, but they are creeping into our other foods in the most unexpected places. Having heard that sugar is the spawn of the devil, we now head towards the 'reduced-sugar' ketchup, only to find it may have been spiked with artificial sweeteners.

5. **Alcohol** – this has been shown to zap our gut flora and cause dysbiosis.

A typical food diary

Here is what a busy London office worker who is watching their weight might eat in one day. This food diary incorporates common patterns and trends that I have noticed when working with corporations and their staff.

Breakfast (on the way to work): Large caffé latte made with skimmed milk

Lunch: pesto and pasta salad

Mid-afternoon: three rice cakes and a diet cola

On getting home: packet of crisps and large glass of white wine while cooking a goat's cheese pizza (marketed as under 500 calories).

This food diary reveals a number of disordered eating patterns that have been fuelled by the messages delivered by popular media on current nutrition trends and outdated science.

• Firstly, the whole food diary contains only small traces of vegetables – the basil in the pesto and a smear of tomatoes and red onions on the pizza. Low levels of vegetables can lead to a low diversity of gut flora and all the problems that go with that – one being difficulty in managing weight. This person may be trying to manage their calories but they are likely to continue to be overweight as well as being tired and in a low mood, catching every cold and suffering from poor skin condition in the process, not to mention feeling constantly hungry.

- Many people drink skimmed milk because we have been told it is 'healthier' for us. We are told that having 2 per cent fat instead of 4 per cent is healthier, however, once the natural fat is extracted from milk it actually becomes a higher-density sugar drink – there is less fat but a higher concentration of lactose from the natural sugar in milk to digest.

- Pasta is often seen as a 'low-fat' meal, but the carbohydrate in pasta turns to sugar quickly when it is broken down by the digestive system. Many of us eat too much wheat – contributing to a monotonous narrow range of foods in our diet, which can lead to a lack of diversity in the gut flora. This office worker is eating wheat for lunch and dinner. Wheat also spikes our fat-storage hormone, insulin, and may lead to a more efficient calorie-extracting microbiome.

- The pizza marketed with a crumble of goat's cheese is rather tasty but still represents an unbalanced meal because 90 per cent of the meal is the base, which is refined flour and so turns to sugar and does all of the above.

- The diet cola contains artificial sweeteners, which have been shown to alter gut flora. The rice cakes are broken down to sugar quickly. The crisps are probably high in fat. The wine may not help your microbiome and could cause dysbiosis.

Where the Western diet is going wrong

Microbiome scientists have been examining the gut bacteria of hunter-gatherers in parts of Africa and South America. Hunter-gatherers are fascinating for microbiome researchers because their diets are thought to have many elements in common with our ancestors. The view is that these people are eating what we are genetically designed to eat rather than the Western, modern diet that most of us eat, which is dominated by farmed foods such as grains and dairy, which only started to become a large part of our diet with the advent of farming just 10,000 years ago. For millions of years before that, we were hunting our own wild meat and fish and picking our own wild fruit and vegetables, nuts and seeds.

Hunter-gatherer tribes' guts teem with an enormously wide variety of bacterial species. Meanwhile those on the Western diet – dominated by one main grain, wheat (rather than a broader range), with a small amount and variety of plant matter, and being high in processed fats, factory-farmed meats and fish, and alcohol – have been shown to have a narrower range of gut flora and a set of non-communicable diseases to go with it. Even rural farming populations in Africa and South America today that eat a broad variety of vegetables and are breast-fed as babies have been shown to have a much better gut bacterial profile than Westerners on the diet described above. So we don't have to turn into full-blown hunter-gatherers to improve our health – we just need to make some significant *Gut Makeover* tweaks to get there.

Here are some of the key areas where our Western diet is currently going wrong.

Low vegetable intake

The British eat on average four pieces of vegetables and fruit per day. The government advises us to eat five portions a day (a portion being about a cupful), however, myriad other sources indicate that we should be eating at least seven portions a day, if not more.

Lack of diversity

How many different plants have you eaten this week? If it's just a handful, the range of your gut flora species could be quite limited, and your health too. The more diverse your intake of plants and wider the range of flora, the better your health and weight. If we want a beautiful microbiome, we need to eat a rainbow of colours and a wide spectrum of varieties. In a recent interview, Jeff Leach, lead researcher of the American Gut project, said he tries to eat 20–30 different plants (vegetables and fruit) per week for a healthy gut microbiome. The greater the diversity of the diet, the greater the diversity of bacteria, and therefore the better your health.

Another concern is that overexposure to particular foods (such as when we are following monotonous diets) can actually lead to us becoming intolerant of those foods, which can lead to further health problems (as mentioned on page 28).

We also need to make sure that some of the vegetables and fruit we eat contain prebiotic fibres. This type of fibre is a big feeder of bacteria in our gut and makes that gut bacteria flourish and bloom. I'll be covering where to find prebiotic fibres in Part 2.

Too much sugar

A high-sugar diet can be detrimental to our microbiome. The reason is that bacteria love sugar, and the non-beneficial ones are likely to get more dense and powerful if we feed them sugar all day leading to dysbiosis. However, if the rest of your digestion is working well, 85 per cent of sugar should have been absorbed before the food reaches the colon.

Too much caffeine

Many of us rely on caffeine from coffee, tea, sports drinks, colas and even green tea to get through the day. We like the quick boost to alertness and energy they seem to give us. There are also antioxidants in coffees and teas, which can offer some benefits to the gut, but a digestive system constantly assaulted with the caffeine accompanying them is unlikely to be operating at its best. This happens because caffeine is a stimulant and can trigger the release of the stress hormones adrenaline and cortisol to get us going. When stress hormones are high, the sympathetic nervous system, known as the 'fight or flight' system, is dominating. This means the parasympathetic nervous system – 'the rest and digest' nervous system, which needs to be switched on to ensure our digestion is working well – may be operating at half mast while the body diverts energy to the more pressing stress situation.

Caffeine also can lead to sugar being tipped from the liver, where it is stored, into the bloodstream. So when you have that first coffee of the morning it doesn't just give you an adrenaline surge but a sugar rush too. To get your digestion in optimal running order during *The Gut Makeover*, it is important to take a break from caffeine.

Overexposure to antibiotics

Antibiotics may kill the bacteria causing you that earache, but they aren't selective about which other bacteria they kill in the body. This means that when you take a course of antibiotics, it is also likely to kill friendly bacteria in your gut. So if the friendly ones take a beating, as well as the lurgies in your ear, you may be left with dysbiosis and a smaller diversity of species in there. Antibiotics have been shown to reduce diversity of the bacteria in the gut in three to four days, with the impact lasting months to years, depending on your diet.

In addition to any antibiotics we take, we may also be being subjected to residues of antibiotics on a low level by consuming farmed fish, meats and dairy, as farmers routinely give prophylactic antibiotics to their livestock.

We have known about the link between antibiotics and weight gain for decades through the observation of farm animals, when farmers noticed that feeding their animals antibiotics had the knock-on, profit-driving effect of making livestock fatter. But what is good for their bottom line isn't helping our waistlines.

I'm not saying never take antibiotics – they can, of course, be life-saving. I'm simply saying there is a time and a place for them and that overexposure could be making us fatter, as well as leading to antibiotic resistance, meaning their ability to save lives is in danger too. So you need to weigh up the pros and cons carefully, and if you do need a course of antibiotics, *The Gut Makeover* is the perfect way to kick-start your microbiome afterwards.

Diet fads and myths

Nutrition is a notoriously confusing and contradictory subject, and many of the health beliefs we have been brought up with are now being challenged by new research. Here we explore the changing nutrition landscape in the early 21st century.

The calorie myth

We now know that the quality of the calories we eat is more important than the numbers; this is because not all calories were created equal. For instance, if you take in 500 calories from drinking cola, it will have a totally different impact on fat deposition to eating the same number of calories from a portion of asparagus and a piece of chicken.

So why is chicken and asparagus so much better? Cola contains high quantities of sugar (usually fructose), and high-sugar diets can upset the balance of the bacteria in your gut, which is also being linked with calorie extraction from food – any food – rising and hunger increasing. In comparison, the chicken contains protein, and protein is the hardest and slowest type of food there is for the body to break down. We burn up to one-third of the calories from chicken just on digesting it. That is called the 'thermogenic' effect of a food. On top of that, the asparagus, besides being a nutrient powerhouse of good vitamins and minerals, contains a particular type of 'prebiotic' fibre which helps beneficial bacteria in your gut proliferate. This diversity of flora could mean less extraction of calories and hunger.

Masses of fast-moving pioneering research has been done in this area. The results indicate that the diversity and balance of this gut bacteria is closely linked with weight. When the range of species within this 1.5kg (3½lb) of bacteria are reduced (such as when we eat a lot of sugar, take antibiotics, eat insufficient vegetables, have foods we are intolerant to or drink a lot of alcohol), we may extract more calories from the food that we are eating.

Thankfully this message is now beginning to be heard and promoted in mainstream medicine. A group led by the previously mentioned cardiologist Dr Aseem Malhotra wrote an editorial in the journal *Open Heart* in 2015: 'Shifting the focus away from calories and emphasising a dietary pattern that focuses on food quality rather than quantity will help to rapidly reduce obesity, related diseases, and cardiovascular risk.'

No one warns us about potential insatiable, uncontrollable, rebound hunger when they recommend a calorie-controlled diet, or how depleted we may become in important vitamins and minerals that are needed for good mental health, which means we may crave food – any food – later on. Nor do they tell us about protecting our immune system and the health of our skin.

To those who nowadays embrace eating quality food and appreciate that being a healthy weight is more than just a calories game, this may all seem obvious. However, I do regularly meet women (and some men) in my clinic who are attached to calories and live every day in a battle with them. More often than not, they are women in my age group and above who, like me, had been conditioned in earlier years to believe this was the right approach. Because it's not working for them, we work together on new approaches – starting with gut health.

Fasting diets

I am often asked about my views on fasting for weight loss and to improve health. More recently, the 5:2 diet of fasting on two days a week (on which you consume just 500 calories if you are a woman and 600 calories if you are a man) has become a popular way to lose weight and improve metabolic markers. This method can be a godsend for some, but it may be a disaster for others. Anecdotally I have come across people who experience immense rebound hunger and weight gain when they stop regular two-days-a-week fasting.

We have to remind ourselves that we are all different, with a unique genetic make-up, and for this reason, one person's meat can be very much another person's poison. There is no one diet in the world that suits all mankind. With *The Gut Makeover* plan, I will encourage you to experiment with foods over these weeks to find out what suits you and doesn't suit you, so you can try to stay healthy for the long term. Personalised nutrition is an exciting way forward.

The sugar crusade

Sugar – the villain that has been on the run for several decades while fat took all the flak – has finally been hunted down and shamed. We've had years of nonsense, demonising all fats and messing around with natural foods to make them supposedly more healthy by extracting their fat content and replacing it with sugar to make them palatable. Reduced-fat yoghurts and frozen yoghurt are prime examples of this approach.

High-sugar diets in animals have been shown to change the balance of the gut flora, with subsequent declines in mental and physical performance, so it's not only the impact of sugar on our weight that we need to worry about. Fructose, the type of sugar found in many fizzy drinks and junk foods, has been shown to induce a leaky gut in animals. However, 'diet' drinks aren't any better. Recent research has indicated that the artificial sweeteners that replace sugar can lead to changes in the flora in the microbiome, which may lead to greater extraction of calories eaten, as well as an increase in type 2 diabetes. This was an early study, and more quality research is needed, but, even so, it is a stark warning, and in my opinion means artificial sweeteners such as aspartame, sucralose and saccharin are best avoided.

Alcohol is also packed with sugar, but as there is no labelling of the ingredients, it is easy to forget that fact.

The problem with high-fat diets

Saturated fats such as coconut oil and butter are now being celebrated for their health benefits, stability, and their lack of adulteration. You can recognise a saturated fat because it is solid at room temperature. They can be heated to higher temperatures before becoming damaged, unlike oils, which are liquid at room temperature.

Fats are an important part of our diets, but high-fat diets have been linked to a reduction in the diversity of gut flora. As we have seen before, diversity is essential to our health and weight. This is why I am weary of those diets where coconut oil is celebrated and slathered on every morsel of food, and dolloped freely into your coffee in the morning (the famous 'bulletproof coffees').

The truth is, if you have too much fat – any fat; it could skew your gut flora and you could gain weight more easily. If you do like to use saturated fats, just watch your quantities.

The Gut Makeover does include fats but not in excessive quantities. Real butter (in the second half of the programme) and virgin olive oil (throughout the four weeks) are my favourite recommendations. Butter contains butyric acid (the fuel needed to build a healthy gut lining), which can also be made by the bacteria in the gut as they ferment vegetable fibres. Butter also contains vitamin A to support the gut lining. Extra virgin olive oil contains plant chemical polyphenols, which can help protect the oil from damage when it is heated. Polyphenols may also help gut flora proliferate.

The Paleolithic (or Paleo) diet

Paleo in its true form is a diet of wild proteins (such as meat, fish, eggs, nuts and seeds) and plants (vegetables and fruits) and is based on an idea of what our original ancestors would have eaten millions of years ago. This means, in theory, eating what the human body evolved to eat.

Eating a natural diet, without the refined flours, sugar, unhealthy fats and artificial sweeteners of the Western diet, can be enormously beneficial to the microbiome – and consequently your weight and health – and my one-month *Gut Makeover* does pay a nod to Paleo. My plan also puts into your diet lots of delicious meat, fish, eggs, nuts, seeds and mountains of vegetables. However, there are two problems with the Paleo diet. One, we are living in a 21st-century industrialised society with very different food access from our ancestors, and two, our protein and plants are, for the major part, not wild, so the nutrient density and quality are far poorer.

With true Paleo diets, all dairy and grains which came into our diet with the advent of farming 10,000 years ago are left out. The argument is that after eating protein and plants for millions of years, our genes have not adapted fast enough over this time frame to digest farmed grains and dairy well. I disagree with the rigidity of the Paleo argument; we now know that our genes are pretty flexible and interact with our environment all the time and are constantly adapting. It has been shown that famines suffered by recent generations can alter genes of children born down the line to help survival in famines, if encountered today. We also know that a healthy microbiome cross talks with our genes, having the potential to switch them on or be silent.

When the Paleo diet is followed using high-quality foods, including wild meats and fish and nutrient-powerhouse organ meats, it can be enormously supportive for some groups of people, in particular those with autoimmune disorders. But I must stress that it is very important to concentrate on the quality aspects of the protein and plants you are eating because in standard Paleo diets the plate is half protein, half vegetables.

The Gut Makeover plan differs from the Paleo in that, while it avoids dairy for part of the programme and gluten, grains and beans for a month while your gut mends, it does not banish these foods for the long term. This is because you are not a caveman and you live in the 21st century, so we need to give you a caveman's microbiome but using the food you have access to in the real world today.

Gluten – to eat or not to eat?

Gluten is often spoken as a bad word, but what is it and where do we find it?

Simply put, gluten is a protein found in certain grains, most commonly wheat, as well as present in trendy grains like spelt. It's in the couscous in that delicious roast vegetable couscous salad we just ate. It's also in the pearl barley enjoyed in that stew at the nice organic cafe, and that semolina pudding in the canteen. We're usually aware that there is gluten in wheat flour, but it's easy to miss it when we're enjoying a home-cooked Sunday roast and only later discover a relative has thickened the gravy with flour. For many people gluten isn't a problem, but increasing numbers of people are finding gluten causes all sorts of issues for their guts.

In the olden days you were either coeliac or non-coeliac. Coeliac disease is a life-threatening autoimmune disorder which is triggered by eating gluten. Gluten causes a tremendous immune reaction in coeliacs, a bit like a fire alarm. A coeliac's immune system does not like gluten and sees it as an invader. After fighting the gluten onslaught for a time, the immune system gives up, gets totally confused and can no longer recognise the difference between gluten and the cells of the small intestine itself. The immune cells then start attacking the gut cells and destroying them. This carpet becomes mowed down and the surface area for absorption of fuel and nutrients isn't there any more, or only parts of it are left. This means the body can no longer absorb food properly and the person becomes ill. If a coeliac continued to eat gluten in this condition, they would die. This is because they can't absorb nutrients and fuel from their food. Just one particle of gluten stuck to a fried chip from the local chip shop which has been cooked in the same oil as the shop's battered fish can ignite a massive immune reaction in a coeliac's gut, destroying parts of the shag pile. Even the slightest, accidental exposure to gluten can set them back.

You can develop and be diagnosed with coeliac disease at any stage of life. It often develops during or shortly after pregnancy, and 20 per cent of newly diagnosed cases are in people over 60. It is not something you are necessarily born with, though there may be a genetic predisposition. Around 95 per cent of coeliacs have either the HLA-DQ2 or HLA-DQ8 genes. If you carry either of these genes you are at risk of developing problems with gluten.

We now know that genes are not, as originally thought, certain fate; we can be born with a particular gene, but it may never get switched on. We also know that our environment can switch on, or silence, particular genes. So for instance, if you are one of the 30 per cent of northern Europeans with the HLA-DQ2 or HLA-DQ8 genes, and you eat gluten for years on end for breakfast, lunch and dinner, washed down with beer made from wheat, your chances of developing coeliac disease are higher than someone with the same genes who eats bread and pasta only occasionally. The other factor is that the wheat we are most exposed to nowadays is the dwarf variety, which has been bred to yield as many tufts as possible without falling down. However, the content of the protein gluten is greater in these plants than in old-fashioned ones such as einkorn wheat or spelt. This means that our exposure to gluten is higher than ever before.

It is estimated that 0.5–1 per cent of European and North American populations have full-blown coeliac disease. However, in contemporary scientific literature, it is estimated that 6–10 per cent of the population is having problems with gluten but do not fit the criteria to be diagnosed coeliac. The term being used to identify and discuss this group is non-coeliac gluten sensitivity (NCGS). However, if you have the HLA-DQ2 or HLA-DQ8 genes you could already be experiencing problems connected with gluten without being coeliac, and these areas are where many people fall.

The New England Journal of Medicine has linked 55 other disorders with eating gluten. These range from rheumatoid arthritis and thyroid disorders to fatigue, anxiety, depression, joint pain, infertility, miscarriages, skin rashes and mouth ulcers. For this reason many people are cutting out gluten-containing foods to see if it makes a difference to their health. Some report that their brain fog disappears; others that the chronic joint pain that they have endured for years miraculously clears up. In some, chronic adult acne disappears or their chronic fatigue clears up. By removing a food that is putting their immune system on low-level constant alert, people often feel more energetic than they have done in years.

Another point to consider is that it is not always the protein gluten that is causing reactivity. In some people it can be other proteins in the wheat kernel. This is why some individuals swear their well-being improves when they give up their usual wheat bread and feel much better on spelt. There is also the possibility that gluten is irritating the gut lining from overexposure; having a pause for a while gives the gut time to heal and allows the gut flora to repopulate.

However, I'm not advising you to swap your usual treats for foods marketed as 'gluten-free'. Whole aisles in supermarkets are appearing dedicated to this topic. Just because a cake or bread says 'gluten-free' does not make it healthy. Read the ingredients list and make your own decisions. When I looked at one mainstream brand of gluten-free bread I identified 33 ingredients, of which many were probably better described as food-like substances. These products are often highly processed, loaded with sugar and made from other grains instead of wheat. For example, you often find rice, maize, buckwheat or soya flour replacing wheat in commercial gluten-free foods. The problem with this is that some people who are sensitive to gluten or wheat may have also lost tolerance of other grains, especially if they are loading their diet with them after quitting gluten.

This is why sometimes coeliacs don't improve on a gluten-free diet – they can be reacting to other grains too so the immune system is constantly being enraged. Before you know it the individual is diagnosed with another autoimmune disorder such as Hashimoto's (where your immune cells attack your thyroid) or rheumatoid arthritis. Autoimmune disorders, unfortunately, often come in clusters if the immune system isn't kept in check.

If you find after this plan that you feel much better not eating gluten, don't turn to commercial gluten-free products. Instead, eat real, home-made foods. You could make a cake with ground almonds instead of flour; you can use a little gem lettuce or chicory leaf as the 'bread' for a sandwich filling. You could also spiralise some chopped courgettes and sauté them in a pan, as a replacement for spaghetti with your bolognaise. Eating real-food replacements is healthier, much tastier and prevents you from subjecting yourself to highly processed alternatives.

Another growing common misconception is that going gluten-free is better for everyone. It isn't. Gluten is not the food of the devil. In fact, certain types of bread such as sourdough could be positively good for your gut flora, and, subsequently, your overall health – as long as you are in the 70 per cent of the population that is likely OK with gluten and has no genetic predisposition to associated problems with the protein.

The Gut Makeover removes gluten from your diet for one month, even if you don't have a sensitivity. Here is the rationale: leaving it out in the short term will encourage you to replace it with many more vegetables in your diet, which will aid micro-biome restoration. This in turn may lead to weight loss as you may extract fewer calories from the food you eat. At the end of the month you may wish to reintroduce gluten into your diet – eating foods like sourdough bread might be helpful for some.

Try to keep a food symptom diary and note any changes in your health for three days during reintroduction. If gluten is a trigger for poor health, you are likely to notice a reaction – from a change in stool pattern and bloating, to mood, skin reactions, brain fog or insomnia. By keeping a diary you may find you discover some key information for managing your health in the long term.

Summary

So this is the science behind why *The Gut Makeover* is good for you and just some of the reasoning as to why certain diet and cooking methods benefit our gut flora and ensure we have a healthy gut lining and good overall health.

In the next part of the book you'll be putting this theory into practice. I'll be encouraging you to make specific changes to your diet for the four weeks of *The Gut Makeover* plan.

PART TWO

The four-week gut makeover

Introduction

This section of the book will explain exactly how the plan works, what you can eat and how you can work this into your day-to-day life. There are helpful strategies for making it work for you, and a 'frequently asked questions' section on pages 128–136 that addresses the most common queries from those following the plan.

The four-week plan basics

Before going into the plan in depth, it's good to get to grips with the basics. Here is an outline of the key principles involved in the one-month gut transformation.

The four weeks are separated into two separate stages. Weeks one and two will focus on **REPAIR**, and then in weeks three and four you'll **REINOCULATE**.

1. Weeks one and two: REPAIR

In this stage you will focus on repairing your gut lining and building a wider array of different types of bacteria through plant variety and volume. The key principles are:

1. **Plants:** Try to get masses of different plants – vegetables, fresh herbs and some fruits – into your meals every day. Think a minimum of seven cups of plants – five as vegetables, two as fruit. In raw weight you are looking for about 750g+ (1½lb+). Aim for 20–30 different varieties per week – imagine a shopping trolley exploding with colour and textures. You might end up spending a bit more on fruit and vegetables than you are used to, but you'll more than make up for it with the money you save on booze and those cappuccinos on the way to work.

2. **Protein:** Buy the best-quality protein you can afford (meat, fish, eggs, nuts, seeds) to include at each meal. On page 119 you will discover how best to do this on a budget. If you're a vegetarian, you can include nuts and seeds as well as eggs for protein during the first fortnight, and see page 88 for details on further vegetarian sources of protein to add in the second fortnight.

3. **Relax and chew properly:** Try not to eat on the run, or 'al desko' (at desks), while working. Take a proper break to eat.

4. **Fast:** Get into the habit of a 12-hour fast between dinner and breakfast, because having a long stretch in the 24-hour cycle without food has been shown to improve the microbiome and increase metabolism. This sounds more dramatic than it is, as most of us do this without thinking, but it is a reminder to avoid late-night snacks or boredom eating after dinner.

5. **Avoid snacking between meals and focus on three structured meals a day.**

Weeks three and four: REINOCULATE

The second half of the plan is the reinoculation stage. It's planting season in your garden; as well as eating all the nourishing foods from weeks one and two, you will focus on introducing the following into your gut:

1. **Prebiotics:** Throughout the course of the four weeks, gradually increase your intake of prebiotic foods. These are foods such as bananas that contain fibres which feed bacteria in the gut and can make friendly species bloom. A full list of these foods can be found on page 116.

2. **Probiotics:** In the third and fourth weeks you'll add probiotic fermented foods to the diet. These foods, usually fermented, contain friendly bacteria which may be missing from your gut, especially useful if you've had antibiotics over the past few years, drunk a lot of alcohol or not been having a very good diet. (For details on these foods, see page 116).

What you can and can't eat on the plan

Alcohol: I'm really sorry to be a killjoy on this one, but if you want to restore your gut to full health, giving up alcohol for a short period is really helpful. It is well documented in gut research that alcohol can damage the mucus in our small intestine and colon and can cause dysbiosis and leaky gut. Have you ever noticed your eczema is worse after a night out drinking? This could be a leaky gut. Or do you suffer loose stools as well as a poor mood the morning after a few drinks? That could be dysbiosis. On *The Gut Makeover*, you are going to give the gut a chance to recover from alcohol.

Caffeine: is a stimulant, which can lead to raised stress hormones and sugar levels in the blood. Lots of caffeine can also lead to the 'rest and digest' part of our nervous system potentially underperforming. *The Gut Makeover* avoids caffeine for one month to help improve your digestive system. See page 73 for tips on weaning yourself off caffeinated drinks.

Sugar and artificial sweeteners: Both sugar and artificial sweeteners such as aspartame, saccharin and sucralose have been linked with suboptimal microbiomes, so for good gut health these are avoided this month.

Dairy (such as milk and cheese) is included but is limited in *The Gut Makeover*. This is because some individuals may have problems digesting it. However, in the 'reinoculate' part of the plan (weeks three and four) it is included in portion-controlled amounts because bacteria in foods such as fermented milk kefir can boost beneficial gut flora, helping weight control, mood balance and the immune system. We'll even include portion-controlled crumbles of Roquefort cheese in weeks three and four (see page 104), for those who can tolerate them, because they are teeming with bacteria to boost gut flora. However, cheese is portion-controlled in this plan because it contains high levels of fat, and a high-fat diet has been shown to be detrimental to a healthy microbiome and to potentially increase caloric extraction from foods. Some fat is good in the diet, but too much could delete all the good work of the bacteria in the cheese. For those of you who suspect you have or have had lactose intolerance diagnosed (usually through a breath test), we will suggest some gut-supporting non-dairy fermented foods.

Digesting lactose

I meet people in my clinic who are fine with the first latte in the morning, but the one after lunch is when all their digestive symptoms start. This may be because the small number of lactase enzymes they produce each day have been used up on breakfast and they can't produce enough for the afternoon latte.

If we eat or drink milk products and don't have enough lactase enzymes to cut up and break down the lactose sugars, they can go through the stomach, the small intestine and end up in the colon undigested. At this point the lactose sugar from the milk – which should have been absorbed through the small intestine into the bloodstream by now – feeds the non-beneficial bacteria, who have a massive party. They tend to produce a lot of gas doing this. We know when this happens – we feel bloated, have wind, and run to the loo with loose stools. It's unpleasant, and makes it difficult to manage weight, mood, skin and immune issues. If you experience these sorts of symptoms, you may find this is why your skin improves when you cut out milk from your diet, or that your mood and weight improves.

Grains, in particular gluten-containing grains such as wheat, rye and spelt, etc., are not included in *The Gut Makeover* because they can irritate the gut lining in sensitive individuals. When we eat a lot of them, we also have less room to eat a wide range of vegetables. So on *The Gut Makeover* you not only leave out the gluten-containing grains but also all other grains, such as rice, oats, and quinoa, so that you can fill their place on the plate with large portions of deliciously prepared vegetables. Grains can then be added back into your diet in the maintenance part of the programme if you like.

Beans and pulses are left out of *The Gut Makeover* because they contain high levels of lectins, which when eaten in high quantities can cause leaky gut, bloating and dysbiosis in some individuals. So for one month the gut is going to have a holiday from them. It is OK to try to return them to your diet on the maintenance part of the programme if your gut lining is in good shape, so you can tolerate them. Pulses do contain prebiotic fibres, which can be beneficial in the long run to your gut flora. I have suggested vegetarians add them back in the diet at the end of the first fortnight, earlier than meat eaters, in order to have more choice of proteins to eat.

Nightshade vegetables (which include potatoes, tomatoes, aubergines, peppers and chillies) are all included in the plan. If you have an interest in gut health and have been reading up about leaky gut, you may have taken the decision to omit nightshade vegetables from your diet because, like pulses, they are higher in lectin proteins than a lot of other vegetables. Of course, if you notice you have difficulties digesting nightshades, leave them out, but in my clinical practice I find it so rare that someone really has a problem with them that I recommend including them so the vitamins, minerals and wide array of plant chemicals in them can be exploited. Cold cooked potatoes feature in the diet so that we can benefit from the resistant starch that develops in them when they cool down. Resistant starch has been shown to help feed beneficial bacteria in the gut.

Fruit: Two pieces (or two cups) of fresh fruit are included in the makeover each day. Fruit is portion-controlled to two pieces daily to keep your sugar intake low while still receiving the benefits from all the fibre, natural plant chemicals, and nutrients in them. Dried fruit is excluded from the diet due to the copious amounts of fructose sugar in it – much more than when fruit is eaten fresh.

Before you start!

Choose when to start

Before you embark on your *Gut Makeover*, schedule a month in your diary and cordon off a period of time you think would work well for you. This plan is designed so that you can continue going about your busy life while following it, and preparation is key to success, but it is important to give yourself the best chance by choosing the optimum time frame to work in, not the most difficult. Make the journey as smooth as you can. Plan to succeed!

Chart your symptoms

Many of us can become focused on weight loss when starting a new style of eating and can lose sight of all the amazing health benefits and small but significant improvements in well-being that accompany eating well.

When I first started working as a nutritional therapist I didn't measure and keep a record of all the small niggles and subsequent improvements in my clients' health. However, I decided to change this after getting blank stares at follow-up meetings when I asked my clients about the bloating, heartburn, constipation, food cravings, skin rashes, swollen ankles, mood swings, cystitis, aching muscles, sneezing fits, stuffy nose and low energy that they had mentioned to me on our first meetings. A month into changing to a gut-supportive diet many clients couldn't remember some of these original ailments, even though they had suffered from them for years. When we feel well, we often can't recall just how bad we felt before. For this reason I now ask everybody to fill out a symptoms questionnaire at each of our meetings. It means that we can measure symptoms and acknowledge improvements as we go along. This can be very motivating for keeping up healthy new habits in the longer term. And, in the rare cases when the score isn't drastically coming down, it enables us to tweak and personalise the diet accordingly.

So, before you start my *Gut Makeover*, please fill out the questionnaire overleaf and add up your score. Be really honest, then shut the book and do not look at it again till after you have filled out the second questionnaire near the end of this book – at the end of your four-week *Gut Makeover*. Then compare overall scores. You may be very surprised.

It can also be interesting to compare scores of your particular problem areas, such as the digestive tract, emotions, skin, etc. *The Gut Makeover* is more than just about losing a few pounds – it's about improving your quality of life all round.

Date: _____

Rate the following symptoms on a scale of 0–5, with 0 being not present at all and 5 being a major symptom:

Emotions

Mood swings _____

Anxiety _____

Overeating _____

Feeling down _____

Trouble falling asleep, early dawn waking or sleeping too much _____

TOTAL _____

Weight

Bingeing (foods or drink) _____

Compulsive eating _____

Cravings _____

TOTAL _____

Digestive

Bloating _____

Acid reflux (heartburn) _____

Loose stools _____

Constipation (less than one stool movement a day) _____

TOTAL _____

Skin

Eczema _____

Psoriasis _____

Acne _____

TOTAL _____

Immune system

Hay fever _____

Asthma _____

Hives _____

Sneezing attacks _____

Stuffy nose _____

Sinus problems _____

Joint aches and pains _____

TOTAL _____

Energy

Fatigue _____

Difficulty getting up in the morning _____

Hyperactivity _____

Lethargy _____

Poor memory _____

Poor concentration _____

TOTAL _____

For women

Premenstrual symptoms _____

Menopausal symptoms _____

TOTAL _____

OVERALL TOTAL SCORE: _____

Measure your weight

If one of your goals from *The Gut Makeover* is to lose weight I suggest you weigh yourself about a week before you start the plan. You may also like to make a note of your waist measurement. Do this before you start reducing your caffeine, alcohol and sugar intake in the pre-plan week. It is best to stand on the scales naked, first thing in the morning. Make a note of the date and time and that this weight is without clothes. This means you can replicate the conditions when you weigh yourself again – halfway through the makeover and again at the end of the four-week plan.

Try not to get on the scales between these points – it can be an unhelpful pressure. There are so many small day-to-day fluctuations and variables to consider, such as how much fluid you have been drinking, your hormone balance, and how often you are having a stool movement. But there is also the matter of your gut flora, and how this is influencing the way in which you are using the calories from the food you are eating and your metabolism.

You'll need a month on the plan for your beneficial gut flora to proliferate and influence your metabolism, and for inflammation to diminish, so let these mechanisms kick in. Some people find weighing in too early demoralising. I've had clients tell me they give themselves a hard time and feel miserable for the whole of the rest of the day if the scales are disappointing. Give your body a proper chance to adapt to the new regime before peeping at the scales. It'll be worth the wait!

Enter your weight and the date the week before you start the makeover:

Weight: _____

Date: _____

Enter your weight and the date two weeks into the makeover:

Weight: _____

Date: _____

Enter your weight and the date on the final day of the makeover:

Weight: _____

Date: _____

CASE STUDY

Clare

Age: 49

Occupation: Journalist

Weight before: 11 stone 5lb (72kg)

Weight after: 10 stone 11lb (68.5kg)

Goals: To lose weight, get more healthy and get rid of my sugar addiction.

Notes: My aim was to have a health MOT. A total reset. I was a complete coffee-head before the makeover – sometimes drinking up to ten cups a day of instant coffee – and I had a massive sugar addiction. I'd buy sweets and chocolate to last the week but they'd be gone in two days. It was starting to worry me. A friend had breast cancer and was treated by a consultant in France who advised her to stay away from sugar.

I'd tried to give up gluten in the past but kept tripping up because, until I did *The Gut Makeover*, I didn't realise that gluten is in almost everything. Even English mustard!

I found I just slotted into the makeover and really enjoyed the plan. I thought it would be hard but it was easy – the replacement concept helped as with a little imagination there really is a replacement for everything. I swapped coffee and tea for rooibos tea. I'd make a shepherd's pie containing ten vegetables with a topping of sweet potatoes, mashed carrots and cauliflower. I swapped spaghetti for spiralised courgettes. And, instead of rice, I'd have a bed of kale.

The banana 'bread' saved me when I wanted something sweet. I did variations with coconut too. I had a handful of rocket salad and a lemony dressing, or a couple of chunks of pineapple to start my meals and help my digestion. I made sure I had two vegetables and fruit at breakfast in a shake – that way I wasn't playing catch up on the vegetable count later in the day. Even my kids got into it! Instead of a Sunday fry-up I made them kale sautéed in a pan, added eggs, crumbled Roquefort on top and served them with sweet potato chips. Delicious – and really filling!

Protein is the key. I now realise that in the past I thought I was eating healthily by having a salad, but because there was no protein it was leading to sugar cravings later on. So I made sure I had protein with every meal. I enjoyed the challenge of adding variation and colour to my plate, like creating a work of art, and used things like mixed peppers, red onions, mango and pomegranate seeds. I also loved the kefir and the green juice.

In the first three days of the makeover I suffered bloating and constipation. Jeannette explained this sometimes happens to people who have a gluten sensitivity while the gut readjusts. I loaded up my shakes with chia seeds or flaxseeds to alleviate this and drank lots of water and it passed. I won't go back to wheat now. And since coming off the plan I have no desire to go back to sugar and caffeine as on the occasions I do as a 'treat' I instantly feel the negative effects on my body.

Benefits: Lost 8lb (3.5kg) and conquered my sugar and caffeine addictions.

Biggest tip: I found my local supermarket selling ready-chopped cauliflower 'couscous', ready-spiralised courgette and ready-chopped pumpkin and squash in a bag.

Kitchen essentials

The *Gut Makeover* plan is simple to follow so you don't need lots of fancy extras, but a few bits of kit are useful. Most of these below you will probably already have in your cupboards.

Knife

Make sure you have a decent chopping knife and regularly sharpen it. You'll be eating a lot more vegetables and fruit probably than normal, so a good knife will make these easier to prepare. Some people shy away from eating vegetables because they say they are too much hassle. I agree, they can be an enormous amount of hassle, but only if your knife is too blunt to prepare them.

A handheld stick blender or stand-alone blender

For 25 years I have used cheap handheld stick blenders. They are fine for making soups and blending fruit into kefir (more on that to come). You can buy them for as little as £5. To make soups and kefir shakes, you will need one of these at the very least. If you have a stand-alone workhorse blender, even better. The more powerful blenders can break down hard substances like blocks of ginger and nuts and seeds into indistinguishable particles without giving up on you.

A set of sturdy, portable, spill-proof containers

You'll need these for your packed lunches. Invest in the ones which are spill-proof (e.g. with clip lids). There's nothing better to put you off taking and making your own food than leaking containers in your bag. Many of the evening meal recipes give good leftovers, which can be taken with you wherever you may be at lunchtime the next day and eaten at room temperature or heated up.

American cup measures

A nest of American cup measures are also needed to measure out your fruits and vegetables and get an idea of portion sizes. They are cheaply sold online, often for less than £5. Alternatively, you can make a fist with your hand to get an idea of a portion of plants.

Modern, safe pressure cooker or slow cooker

People sometimes shy away from slow-cooked foods, saying they are worried that the vitamins and minerals are boiled out of the vegetables and meat cooking this way. Yes, that would be the case if you boiled them in water, then threw the water away. However, with stews, you eat all the liquid containing these nutrients too. Many of the micronutrients in meat and bones are very important for building a strong gut lining – for instance, the amino acids in meats are needed for growth and repair of the gut lining. The micro minerals such as zinc, vitamin A, and the omega-3 essential fatty acids found in grass-fed and wild animals all support a healthy gut lining too.

Foods that are cooked in a pressure cooker, or slow-cooked for long hours on the stove or in an oven are easier to digest. This includes beans which can be difficult to digest if not cooked really well. On the maintenance part of the plan, if you decide to reintroduce pulses and beans, cooking them thoroughly is essential to good digestion. Many of us don't have much time for doing this, but a slow cooker is a great option – you can chop up your veg and meat and leave it to bubble away all day. However, my life was transformed when my mother-in-law gifted me with a pressure cooker. These allow you to enjoy the benefits of slow cooking in no time at all. Pressure cookers have a poor image – I associated them with a lot of rattling and steam when I was a kid. Modern, safe pressure cookers and slow cookers are great investments for your health and come in a variety of sizes and prices, but both are generally fairly inexpensive.

Preparation week

Alcohol, caffeine, artificial sweeteners and sugar may all adversely impact your gut flora and the condition of your gut lining. We want to give your digestive system a break from these substances during *The Gut Makeover* so your gut lining can mend and your flora repopulate. Remember that the plan is only four weeks short. So if you normally drink alcohol and/or coffee it means you can still enjoy those for the other 48 out of 52 weeks of the year, but during these four short weeks they are left out.

However, going cold turkey – particularly from caffeine – can create tiredness and headaches so, to make the plan easier, try to come off them slowly before the makeover month to minimise the impact. I recommend starting to cut down on alcohol and caffeine as well as any diet drinks containing artificial sweeteners such as aspartame or sugar gradually in the week before *The Gut Makeover*.

Start by cutting down on coffee or tea (including green tea, which contains some caffeine). For example, if you usually have a two-shot latte daily, reduce it to one-shot for a couple of days, then none. Colas and diet colas which also contain caffeine should also be reduced slowly.

Experiment with alternatives. For example, if you like black tea, substitute it for rooibos (also known as redbush tea), which doesn't contain caffeine, or other herbal teas. One option may be to boil a few slices of fresh ginger in water for ten minutes, then strain the liquid as a tea. It smells delicious and warming, and can be particularly welcoming when you open a hot flask of it on a cold day. Ginger is anti-inflammatory; like aspirin and ibuprofen, it is a COX-2 inhibitor for pain relief but it comes without the risks of damaging the stomach lining. I like to think of it like a nice shot of calm – to ease up aches and pains.

Do note that 'decaffeinated' teas and coffees usually still contain a small amount of caffeine so they aren't suitable for the plan. However, you might choose to use them to help you slowly transition off these drinks and replace them with healthier alternatives. However, once into the plan, I recommend not having decaffeinated drinks as they have usually been highly processed, and we're aiming to focus on unprocessed foods for the month.

I have seen a run of clients who when we met were drinking diet cola all day. Several have described it as an 'addiction'. We usually work on reducing the intake gradually (to avoid the caffeine-withdrawal headaches). So if they are on six a day, I'd get them to reduce by one a day, replacing each drink with alternative options. Good old plain water is great, preferably filtered as it's more environmentally friendly than bottled and you don't risk the problem of leached plastics in your drink.

A lot of the sugar we have each week comes from liquid – often without our realising it. The biggest culprits are often fresh fruit juices that we buy in the fridge section of the supermarket. However, a third of the carton is often sugar (natural fructose sugar). You can get plenty of vitamins and minerals from fruit without drinking buckets of it juiced. If you drink a glass of juice every day, try watering it down over a few days, and then switching to a glass of water in the morning with a peeled orange instead or a chopped-up piece of fruit with the fibre still in it for your vitamins.

If you are a daily wine or beer drinker, switch to smaller glass sizes. If you're a white wine drinker you could dilute it with fizzy water to become a spritzer. If you're a red wine drinker you could start imposing portion control by buying airline-size quarter bottles (187ml/6½fl oz). Many supermarkets now sell them and it means less temptation than an open 750ml (1⅓-pint) bottle.

Cutting out alcohol can seem off-putting at first, especially if you usually have alcohol every day to wind down, or to cushion nerves at social functions when you are meeting new people. Feedback from *Gut Makeover* participants is that the idea of cutting out booze was far more scary than actually doing it, and the benefits more than made up for it. They also said they started enjoying their food more and loved waking up at weekends without a hangover.

Many of us drink more alcohol than is good for us, and lots of alcohol is like pouring weed killer on our gut bacteria. So while you're promoting abundance and diversity of your gut bacteria over this month, it's important not to have the odd sneaky drink. In terms of building a healthy gut lining and a wide range of bacteria so that you build your resilience for the future, pausing alcohol for 4 out of 52 weeks this year could be one of the best things you do for your overall health.

Aim by the end of this pre-week to have removed drinks containing alcohol, caffeine, sugar and artificial sweeteners from your diet altogether (see page 58), so that you are ready to hit the ground running on day one of *The Gut Makeover*.

Celia

Age: 48

Occupation: Full-time parent and volunteer

Weight before: 12 stone (76kg)

Weight after: 11 stone 5lb (72kg)

Goals: Lose weight, have more energy throughout the day and upgrade my diet for better health.

Notes: After the first week I was amazed how easy it all became. I did *The Gut Makeover* at the same time as three friends, and we haven't been comparing horror stories, we've been comparing success stories. This plan is not about deprivation, it's about abundance.

When you go off processed foods it's interesting what happens to your taste buds. I noticed quickly things were becoming too sweet. Soon your taste buds become keener and you appreciate food more. In the second week, I put a bit of bought mayonnaise on something. I thought, 'This tastes kind of fake and bizarre.'

I love drinking – cocktails, wine, Champagne – but I have not missed pausing alcohol one single bit. Having been to several parties with alcohol flowing freely I have been happy to be there with my sparkling mineral water or coconut water – as long as I could drink it from a wine glass!

A challenge for me was rethinking breakfast. In the past it was easy to reach for toast and use it as a vehicle for jam.

With *The Gut Makeover* I have been making omelettes using leftovers in them (such as roast vegetables), and sometimes I'd eat half for breakfast warm, and half for lunch, cold. Breakfast is something you have to crack at the beginning. You need to know what you will do the night before. You need to plan.

After *The Gut Makeover* I am taking more pride in what I eat. I hadn't realised what a rut I was in. Before I was having too much sugar, white carbs and caffeine. I am very grateful for the introduction to this way of eating, and will take elements from it away – such as eating more veg and a greater variety of it. I no longer snack, and I'm more conscious of chewing my food properly. The evening meals on the plan have been so good that my husband didn't even know he'd been eating *Gut Makeover* meals for a week until a friend told him!

Benefits: I've dropped a dress size, don't have afternoon dips in my energy any more and I've lost my sweet tooth. I am eating a better quality diet and so is the rest of the family. I started seeing the benefits in the first five days.

Biggest tips: Get through the first week and don't give up. Don't underestimate the withdrawal symptoms from caffeine and sugar, but it does get so much better so quickly. To keep yourself interested in the food, treat yourself to big tastes, like fish sauce, tamari, mustard and balsamic vinegar. Use Asian and Indian cuisine and include coconut milk for a creamy taste. Don't bland yourself out.

Keep an eye out for hidden sugars

Cutting out sugar and sweeteners might sound simple, but it's actually far more complex than just looking for the word 'sugar' on the packaging. To wean yourself off the sweet stuff in drinks during the pre-week, and in both food and drinks, during the four-week *Gut Makeover*, you'll need to become literate in the many different names that sugar and sweeteners can come under. Once you're familiar with these terms, you may be surprised at how many of the products in your cupboards contain secret sugars.

Here are just some of the many names to look out for on labels representing sugar or sugar substitutes to avoid

- HFCS (high-fructose corn syrup)
- Fructose
- Fruit juice concentrate
- Glucose
- Glucose syrup
- Galactose
- Granulated white sugar
- Brown sugar
- High maltose corn syrup
- Maltodextrin
- Muscovado
- Rice syrup
- Hydrogenated starch hydrolysates
- Mannitol
- Maltitol
- Treacle

- Invert sugar
- Artificial sweeteners (e.g. sucralose, aspartame and saccharin)
- Xylitol
- Agave syrup
- Stevia
- Coconut sugar
- Sorbitol
- Erythritol
- Dextrose
- Sucrose

Sugars to use extremely sparingly in this plan and during maintenance

- **Honey:** This is a natural prebiotic substance that will feed the beneficial bacteria in the gut. Honey is sweeter than sugar, so you need very little. It is a good option to include in your cooking in small treat portions. If you can afford it, choose raw honey, which has undergone less processing than regular honey so contains more enzymes, which are better for your digestion. Use in minuscule amounts during the plan.
- **Maple syrup:** This is digested quickly so should only be used sparingly. It contains trace minerals such as manganese (which is needed to make energy in the body) and zinc (which is good for the skin). Make sure you use an unadulterated pure form (i.e. not one mixed with corn syrup). This can be added to your diet in the maintenance part of the programme.

Weeks one and two:
REPAIR

You've cut out the bad stuff in the preparation week – the hard bit is over – now it's time to start putting the good stuff into your diet. I've already covered the basics of this plan to repair your gut on page 56 but here is the detail.

Rethink your plate

We've discussed in Part 1 the problems with the Western diet's reliance on gluten and sugar, and how these foods can cause problems in the body. But, on a practical level, how can you actually eat without relying on these foods? What does breakfast without toast or cereal look like? What on earth is lunch if you can't eat sandwiches any more – not even posh ones like ciabatta rolls or chicken tikka wraps? What does dinner look like if you can no longer eat a staple like pasta?

The first thing we need to question is if breakfast, lunch or dinner really need any cereal, bread or pasta in them at all. On the most basic level, **look at your plate – it should ideally be two-thirds plants, one-third protein.**

Eat a large quantity and variety of plants

You need to crowd out the gluten and other grains plus sugar in your diet with tonnes of plant matter – vegetables, fresh herbs and fruit – which are needed to promote a healthy gut lining and microbiome. **Aim to eat at least seven cupfuls of plants per day instead: five as vegetables, two as fruit.**

For measuring, we are talking about raw weight when chopped. If you don't have a cup in front of you, think about what 750g+ (1½lb+) of vegetables looks like (this is the pre-cooked weight). Another way to visualise portions is to make a fist with your hand and imagine seven vegetables and fruit to the volume of seven fists. On the first day, when planning your meals, you could chop up your plants into measuring cups so you can see what these portion sizes look like. Once you know, you won't have to do this every day, but it does help you visualise it.

For a diverse microbiome for good health, you need a varied diet. **Try to aim to eat between 20 and 30 different varieties of vegetables (including herbs) and some fruits per week.** But on a practical level how do you do this?

Let's imagine an office worker on a normal working day. Let's call her Jenny. At lunchtime she goes into her regular food shop. She knows she needs to avoid gluten, so her usual sandwich is not an option. And she has the aim of getting two cupfuls of vegetables into her diet this lunchtime. Suddenly she's scanning the shelves for a big bowl of salad as a main meal – for example, going for a tuna Niçoise salad, which includes a big pile of green leaves, tomatoes, onions, a few olives, some satiating protein as tuna and boiled egg, and a lemony dressing. The fact she's not eating bread means she has more room, both on her imaginary plate and appetite-wise, for plants to the volume size of two American cups.

After this, a colleague offers her a biscuit. Instead, she eats an apple. This means she has clocked up another portion of plant material. By having the apple, instead of a biscuit, she is crowding out the higher sugar/gluten experience. She also has to chew the apple more slowly, which makes her feel fuller, and it contains pectin, which is a prebiotic and good for her gut flora.

When Jenny gets home she has a bolognaise which she cooked at the weekend and defrosted before going to work. Instead of filling the bottom half of her plate with a big pile of white spaghetti, she spiralises two courgettes and pan-fries them in a tablespoon of olive oil till soft. She slides them onto the plate and piles the bolognaise sauce on top. Two whole courgettes – that's another two cup sizes of plants that have just crowded out the equivalent in volume of gluten which would have been found if she'd had the usual pasta. White pasta is broken down into sugar in the digestive tract quickly, so this is actually a double whammy. It's a gluten and sugar crowd out.

Having seen Jenny's lunch and evening meal, she has clocked up five portions of plants. So I'll now talk about breakfast, because now you've seen the rest of the day, you'll understand why getting in two portions of plants at breakfast is so important. Miss that slot and it's hard to catch up the rest of the day.

So back on our cupfuls, Jenny has a cup full of blueberries, followed by two eggs scrambled with a cup of spinach, which has been melted in the pan with a teaspoon of extra virgin olive oil or a knob of ghee or butter. (Extra virgin olive oil contains polyphenols to help gut flora proliferate, and ghee and butter contain nutrients for a healthy gut lining.) This breakfast takes three minutes to prepare and contains two portions of plants.

Some days Jenny might just tip some leftover roasted vegetables into a pan with her scrambled eggs – such as sweet potatoes, peppers and spinach. Other days she makes a shake in a blender with a cup of uncooked kale, 2cm (¾in) of fresh ginger, a few mint leaves, a squeeze of lemon, an orange with all the pith and a large handful of almonds which have been soaked overnight. On these days she's over two portions of plants before she's even left the house – and this breakfast took just a couple of minutes to make.

In one day Jenny reaches seven portions of plants and feels nicely full after each meal. She avoids high levels of sugar and cuts out gluten and other grains such as rice, oats, quinoa, and processed soya altogether. Her intestines have an opportunity to diversify flora populations due to variety of diet, which also helps her weight and health. And if she had previously had any sign of leaky gut, the main potential irritants have been removed to help her gut heal.

Breakfast

If you don't feel hungry in the morning, I suggest having a liquid breakfast. No, this doesn't involve alcohol! A meal you drink can be easier to consume in sips sometimes than full-on food that you have to chew. See the recipe section for liquid breakfasts – some are portable, and you may be able to have your liquid breakfast later in the morning when you do get hungry. If this is the case, make sure you have a nice four-and-a-half- to five-hour gap till lunch, and consequently till dinner, then aim for a 12-hour fast overnight till the next meal.

Clementine

Age: 40

Occupation: Book editor

Weight before: 10 stone 6lb (66kg)

Weight after: 9 stone 12lb (62.5kg)

Goals: I had put on weight in the last year and wanted to lose that. I would normally never do a 'diet', but I had read the Giulia Enders book on new gut science called *Gut*, so I was interested to try the practical *Gut Makeover*.

Notes: Usually I eat snacks mid-morning and then at 4pm I'm on biscuits and cakes if they are around. I have a weak spot for salami. In the summer I was in France and was having on average two glasses of wine every evening. When I got back, a friend suggested doing *The Gut Makeover*, so we did it together.

The good thing is I did not have the feeling of being on a 'diet'. It did not feel restricted and I was never hungry. The feeling of satiety is very different with this vegetable-rich diet to a grain one. With the *Gut Makeover* foods I feel full, but never heavy, which is the sensation I feel with grains. In the first couple of days I had the worst headache.

I enjoyed having seven vegetables and fruit every day and aiming for 30 varieties a week. It was pretty easy to do, especially when you make a big salad with parsley, toma-toes, artichokes, leeks and you just keep going. I loved the nut cake or banana bread for breakfast with some green gunge. And it was really good having three real meals a day and no snacking.

I have been to parties this month. I went to a friend's 40th birthday and I told them I would be the first on the dance floor. The best thing about going to a party and just drinking water is that you get well hydrated then wake up the next day and can be on good form on three hours' sleep!

Doing *The Gut Makeover* has been really good for me. It brought more awareness of how eating makes me feel. It was a great experience.

Benefits: I lost 8lb (3.5kg), slept better and felt more energetic. The biggest thing for me was no pre-menstrual tension. I used to get bloated, have water retention, constipation, and mood swings but this month I had none of that.

Biggest tip: If you go overboard in the holidays, this is a good way to reframe your eating into a good pattern again. I am going to go back to this plan every six months.

Improve your digestion with bitter leaves and other foods

It always amazes me how many practices found in cultural cooking unwittingly provide significant health benefits. Ever been to France and wondered why they go to the trouble of opening the meal with chicory and grapefruit salad, or a simple pile of bitter leaves with a dressing of extra virgin olive oil and freshly squeezed lemon? Have you enjoyed salads for starters in Italy made of sharp, bitter radicchio or rocket leaves? When we chew food thoroughly hydrochloric acid release is triggered in the stomach, which we need in order to break down our food properly. But chewing bitter leaves such as rocket, chicory or radicchio, also triggers stomach-acid release, aiding digestion further. Get into the habit of having some bitter leaves and a vinaigrette dressing whenever you can – either as a starter, a side salad or even beefed up into a main meal. By adding them as side salads and starters your digestion may be improved, and you'll also clock up extra vegetable portions to benefit your gut, weight and health.

Sharp citrus fruits, such as lemon or grapefruit juice are also triggers of stomach-acid production, so the lemon, grapefruit and even oranges will also help you have enough stomach acid to do a good job of breaking down your food before it goes on to the intestines. Another trick is to eat fresh (not cooked) pine-apple or papaya with your starters or main meals as they contain natural plant enzymes, a kind of chemical scissors, which help break down and make your overall meal easier to digest. Often foods work synergistically together for optimum absorption of nutrients. Another important nutrient is iron. To absorb iron well, you need to combine it with food containing vitamin C, which is why it's a good idea to cut up an orange (vitamin C) alongside your breakfast egg (iron), or squeeze lemon juice onto your green-leaf salads.

In Middle Eastern cooking, carrot sticks are often offered with hummus; a benefit being that eating hummus, which is made with chickpeas mixed with olive oil, provides the fat (oil) that helps you absorb the vitamin A from the carrots to build a strong gut lining.

Include good-quality protein

To repair your gut lining throughout the four weeks, **eat protein from animals from the best sources you can access and afford.** The antibiotic load should be less from animals which have been reared organically, and should not be present at all in wild animals. Less antibiotics in them means less antibiotic residues in you. This, in turn, should mean a healthier microbiome (as antibiotics kill gut flora) and less fat storage and weight gain. You need to eat a significant amount of protein with each meal so you feel full up and so it will provide the building blocks for a healthy gut lining. Quality sources of protein with every meal are also important to help you make it from one meal to the next without snacking. Having enough protein with each meal may be the difference between you sticking with *The Gut Makeover* and not sticking with it. The main *Gut Makeover* protein sources are: meat, fish and seafood, nuts and seeds, and eggs.

It is estimated that the average adult needs 45g (1.5oz) – 56g (2oz) of protein per day. The grams of protein are the numbers of protein in the food, not the overall weight of the food itself, such as an egg or piece of chicken. For example, a large egg has around 7g (⅓oz) of protein and a piece of chicken or fish (100g/3½oz) has an average of 20g (⅔oz). This would mean you need a piece of chicken the size of a pack of playing cards, or a piece of fish the size of a cheque book, as well as an egg to have enough to fill you up properly and meet your daily needs. The daily recommended Reference Nutrient Intake (RNI) of protein is 0.75g per kilogram of your weight if you want to work it out for yourself. Another important point is that you may need even more protein than average if you are experiencing a stressful life-style or exercise a lot. In these cases you are likely to need more protein than the average individual – maybe as much as double. Heavy exercisers have higher protein needs than average to repair and build muscles. Hormones are made from protein, so when we are producing copious amounts of adrenaline and cortisol stress hormones all day long, the raw materials from the protein are used to keep making the stress hormones. This can leave us short of amino acids for making thyroid hormones (needed to balance our weight) and sex hormones (to make us fertile). If you are a particularly stressed individual, and therefore needing to consume more than the average 45g – 56g (2oz) protein a day, it is worth considering organic or wild meats and fish wherever possible, as these are more anti-inflammatory and healthful than factory-farmed ones.

For gut repair, **incorporate organ meats into your diet once or twice a week**. Meats such as chicken livers, ox hearts and kidneys are inexpensive nutrient powerhouses that build healthy gut linings. If you are vegetarian or don't like organ meats, you can get the vitamin A needed for building your gut lining from the yolk in eggs. (Contemporary research challenges the cholesterol hypothesis most people associate with these foods; sugar and white carbs are now believed to be the bigger problem with heart disease.) Butter will be added back into your meals in the next stage of the plan.

Vegetarians and protein

In the first fortnight vegetarian sources of protein are eggs, nuts and seeds. In order to get an idea of portion sizes let's look at how you might get your 45–56g of protein a day.

So, on one day you could have two eggs (14g protein), and 100g of pumpkin seeds which contain about 32g of protein. The pumpkin seeds could be zoomed up in a morning shake, sprinkled on soups and salads, and scattered on roast vegetables and toasted.

Another example might be walnuts. You would need about one American cup size of them (125g) to gain 30g protein in one day. Again the nuts can be scattered on food throughout your meals.

Try to vary your selection of nuts and seeds as much as possible to broaden your range of types of proteins you eat. Variety is important to our gut health.

In the second half of the makeover, vegetarians can introduce pulses such as lentils and beans, so that there are more protein options to choose from. For instance, half a tin of chickpeas (200g) would give you about 15g of protein. A half tin of red kidney beans about 11g.

You can quickly check the protein content (as well as other nutrients) of many foods here: http://nutritiondata.self.com

Think colourful

Once you get used to thinking about your meals in terms of a portion of protein along with piles of brightly coloured vegetables, it should become an automatic style of planning and eating. When shopping try to arrive at the checkout with the most colourful trolley in the queue.

Choose non-dairy fats in the first fortnight

Use non-dairy fats, such as extra virgin olive oil, to cook and make dressings. Extra virgin olive oil is a cornerstone of *The Gut Makeover*; its virgin and extra-virgin forms contain particular plant chemicals called polyphenols, which have been linked with boosting bacteria in the gut. They also have anti-inflammatory properties and taste delicious. Coconut oil is also an option for cooking and is an anti-inflammatory. For more on using fats and oils during the plan, see page 110.

Chew properly and relax

Move away from your desk and computer screen, and switch off your phone when eating. **Try to chew each mouthful 20 times to stimulate the production of stomach acid and enzymes** to help digestion and absorption of your food, and to avoid dysbiosis in the colon.

Chewing properly improves digestion and the absorption of the foods you eat for a knock-on impact on your health and weight. It may also ease digestive complaints such as heartburn, burping, stomach pains, abdominal bloating, constipation or loose stools, and embarrassing wind.

For the *Gut Makeover* plan, it is especially essential to chew properly and relax when eating as you are upping the protein in your diet. As mentioned before, protein requires the body to use more energy to break it down than any other macronutrient, and this helps weight management. Therefore you need plenty of stomach acid and enzymes for the breakdown to happen well. Chewing repeatedly stimulates the production of both the acid and the enzymes. Chewing also stimulates the renewal of cells in the gut lining – which you need for a healthy shag-pile carpet (villi) in there to help with nutrient absorption.

I'm a great believer in chewing every mouthful of food 20 times – though I admit it is still a challenge. I have been doing this for about three years and I still have to remind myself to do it.

So how does chewing 20 times help you manage your weight? Some people say to me that bolting their food and the thought of it going through the digestive system out the other end undigested is a good thing. But we have already learnt how damaging un-digested food can be to the intestinal lining – triggering leaky gut, inflammation and dysbiosis, which may lead to extracting more calories from the food we eat.

But another big reason why chewing properly helps us to manage our weight is because we can identify when we feel full and so are less likely to overeat. It takes about 20 minutes for our satiety hormones to kick in after eating, so imagine you've bolted a sandwich walking along the street to an appointment you have to get to in a hurry. You scoffed the lot in five minutes. Straight after the sandwich you may already be thinking how you fancy a bag of crisps, and, you know you shouldn't, but a Mars would really do the trick too. So you pop into a newsagent and bolt those too. You're still within the 20-minute window. You are now ready for a bucket of latte (there's some special offer on: 20p more for a supersize), which you take to your appointment with you, and start slurping during your meeting. None of these foodstuffs, even when eaten in a relaxed setting and chewed slowly, would be beneficial for your gut, but we're talking about *how* this lunch is eaten rather than *what* is in it at this stage. Because this is the thing: I wonder if you would even get to the Mars bar or the latte if you ate the sandwich and crisps while chewing repeatedly and relaxing.

Let's rewind to the place where you grab the sandwich, and say you also pick up the crisps, the Mars bar and a latte on the way out. You go to a park bench and open your plastic bag. You start to chew every mouthful of your sandwich 20 times. You start to really taste the prawns and the mayonnaise and become aware of the texture and sponginess of the 50/50 bread. You pause between mouthfuls. It takes you at least 10 minutes to eat the sandwich. After that, you pause for five minutes before you spend another five minutes eating the bag of crisps. Now we're up to the 20-minute mark and the satiety hormones kick in, telling your brain your stomach is full. You're now facing the Mars bar and latte, regretting you ever bought them, and certainly not needing them.

The reason why we need to try to engineer a relaxing setting to eat in is obvious from a physiological perspective, but often completely lost in the noise of fad diets. So here we go . . .

I've already briefly touched on the two sides of the nervous system: the sympathetic nervous system (often called 'fight or flight') and the parasympathetic nervous system (often referred to as the 'rest and digest' system). The way these two systems interact is simple: when the fight-or-flight nervous system is dominating, the rest-and-digest system goes on the back burner. This means that if we're wolfing down that sandwich at our desk in mouthfuls, between answering urgent emails, the fight-or-flight nervous system is dominant.

Fight or flight is meant to be just for that – running from extreme danger, such as a wild animal which is going to kill you for its dinner. When we're in fight or flight, the nervous system prioritises sending energy to our brain and into our muscles to run as fast as possible. It says, 'I'm not going to digest the last meal eaten. That can sit in the stomach and wait for my attention later.' So when you eat in a stressed state, not only might the food not have been chewed properly because you were wolfing it down but the digestive enzymes and stomach acid needed to break the food down further are also compromised. This means there will be more food in the digestive tract which is only partially digested. And, as we've seen before, undigested food particles can lead to permeability issues and inflammation, as well as dysbiosis, which can skew your metabolism and your immune and nervous systems.

So find a quiet spot away from your emails, your texts and your computer, and **eat in a relaxed manner**. And if you suffer from digestive issues which lead to your immune system becoming a mess, the time you'll have off work for illness, and your overall reduced productivity could add up to hundreds of hours more than a small 20-minute window in each working day to eat properly.

CASE STUDY

Rachel

Age: 48

Occupation: Interior designer

Weight before: 9 stone (57kg)

Weight after: 8 stone (51kg)

Goals: This was about me and my well-being in an everyday scenario. It was a chance to rebalance and improve digestive issues (bloating and cramping).

Notes: In the first week I was very busy with work, and travelling. The 12-hour overnight fast was not possible, so I just said to myself for that week that's how it has to be. The first few days were an endurance. I had been on holiday the week before, and read the makeover when I got back and was starting the programme on week one without much prep.

I was surprised by the size of headache I had in the first week, but I sustained myself by spoiling myself through food – good stews or a good steak, squid or salmon, and piles of healthy vegetables. I would never expect you could eat so well and lose weight. I really practised having pineapple or lemony/lime foods before eating the main meal and trying to slow down chewing. It all became easy and pleasurable.

I was very busy with work over these weeks, and in the first week travelling, but when things were hard I went and enjoyed what I was eating.

It was really good. It was an indulgence for me to do this programme. *The Gut Makeover* has put a lot of things on my radar and reinspired my cooking and enjoyment of fresh foods.

Benefits: On weeks two and three I felt a real clarity of focus and concentration. I slept really well. My digestive symptoms of bloating – which I have had my whole life – disappeared. I feel more in touch with my feelings, and I have more energy. I lost 1 stone (6kg), and the biggest chunk of that was between weeks two and three, but the really big part of this is not the weight, it is the lifestyle.

Biggest tip: Really focus, prepare and read the book carefully and absorb it before you get started. Build in time for the pre-prep – it will help your first week go well.

Replace quick cooking methods, with slow – or at least slow-style – ones . . .

This one is very simple: include stewed meats and casseroles in your cooking often. Meat that has been well cooked is easier to digest and absorb nutrients from. There is less work for your stomach acid and those natural scissor cutters, your digestive enzymes, to do.

Imagine you cook a steak, but sadly it's tough as old boots. You're going to have to do a hell of a lot of chewing. But that is just the first part of it. Your stomach acid and digestive enzymes will have their work cut out too. If you haven't managed to chew food thoroughly, and your digestion isn't working optimally, undigested particles of your steak could be reaching your colon and causing dysbiosis.

By contrast, imagine you had a Moroccan lamb tagine with almonds and vegetables that had been slowly stewed for several hours. You can do this either in a casserole dish in the oven, or a pot over the stove, or in a slow cooker. Or you could use a safe, modern-day pressure cooker for 30 minutes. The meat would be extremely tender, as would the vegetables. The cooked nuts would also be easier to digest and break down than raw nuts. (If you ever find nuts difficult to digest, I recommend either soaking them overnight before grinding them into your breakfast shake or stewing them.)

If your meats and nuts are tender and snipped up into tiny particles by your digestive enzymes, the nutrients can glide through your gut lining into your bloodstream and charge you with goodness. It also means that your gut flora won't be bombarded with undigested food, which could cause bloating, gas and possibly weight gain.

Fast overnight

Aim for a 12-hour overnight fast between dinner and breakfast. If you eat breakfast regularly at 7am, the last morsel of food passing your lips in the evening would be at 7pm. Or if you eat breakfast at 9am, don't eat anything after 9pm.

After this last meal of the day has been digested and absorbed during sleep, your body breaks down stored sugars in the liver to power its metabolic functions overnight. When this stored sugar in the liver is used up, the body starts breaking down stored fat and turning it into energy to function. Even when we are asleep we need fuel to power all our organs. Well, that has been the main explanation till now. The other mechanism at play with an overnight fast is it most likely resets your microbiome, which in turn has a positive impact on your weight and health. Last year, a significant study from the Salk Institute in California showed that when mice were only allowed an eight-hour window in which to eat they absorbed less calories from their food (proven by high levels of particular sugars in their poo – xylose and galactose – meaning they hadn't absorbed them) than mice who ate their food supplies round the clock. The eight-hour access group also had more diversity of bacterial species in their guts than the ad lib groups. The authors concluded that restricting the feeding window in a 24-hour period influences the microbiome, which in turn impacts metabolism.

Many of us can't limit eating to an eight-hour window, but twelve may be practically possible and beneficial, and even sustainable long term.

Summary: What to eat in weeks one and two

- Get as much variety of plants – vegetables and fresh herbs, and some fruits – into your meals as possible. Think a minimum of seven cupfuls of plants daily – five as vegetables, two as fruit – and aim for at least 20–30 varieties per week. Your fridge should be an explosion of colour and textures. The wider the variety of plants, the wider the diversity of flora in the gut, and the better your health.
- Include proteins (such as meats, fish, eggs, nuts and seeds) with each meal.
- Choose non-dairy fats – mainly extra virgin olive oil – to cook and make dressings. Coconut oil is also an option for cooking.
- Make time to eat, relax and chew properly.
- Avoid snacking between meals and try to leave a 12-hour gap between dinner and breakfast the next morning.

Weeks three and four:
REINOCULATE

ongratulations! After two weeks, you may have dropped a few pounds already. You may have more energy and friends might be saying you look younger and your tummy is flatter. Some *Gut Makeover* participants describe a few days into the plan as 'a whole new way of life' – never going hungry; no counting calories; three delicious meals a day. Many say their appetite has reduced and they have adjusted protein sizes accordingly. They aren't missing alcohol or sugar. They can't believe that they aren't hungry between meals, and that, after initial adjustments and planning, new habits have now formed.

Now this is the point at which I suggest you put your foot on the gut bacteria accelerator. So far you've focused a lot on gut repair and boosting the variety of bugs in your gut by eating at least 20–30 varieties of plants a week, if not more. (One recent *Gut Makeover* participant got up to 67 in a week!) Now it's time to plant some new friendly species of specific bugs into the gut, for a bit more va va voom. These will be introduced through fermented foods. This is the reinoculate stage.

Step up 'prebiotic' vegetables and fruits

Prebiotic foods are those containing certain materials which cannot be broken down in the upper digestive system. When they reach the colon, they provide food for other bacteria. When these prebiotic fibres are combined with probiotic foods, they can boost your flora even more.

On page 116 you will find a list of fruit and vegetables, including bananas, apples, asparagus, leeks, onions, garlic and cold potatoes, all of which contain prebiotic fibres. You may have been including some of these foods in the first fortnight of the plan without really even thinking about it. In weeks three and four, try to focus a little more on stepping these up – bit by bit. It is best to build up your intake of prebiotic plants gradually to avoid wind; start with half a banana, or a small banana each day, and go from there.

Prebiotic foods are attracting a lot of research attention, and are being touted as potentially being even more important than probiotic fermented foods for their health benefits. The thinking is that you can boost your good bacteria in the gut just through increasing your prebiotic foods. They are also good for weight loss because the fibre in them makes us feel full for a long time. This is worth bearing in mind if you can't tolerate probiotic fermented dairy or miso foods.

Cold potatoes may sound like an odd prebiotic, but when potatoes cool down after cooking they form a type of fibre in them called resistant starch. This starch can't be digested anywhere else except the colon. It can make you feel full up as it stays in the digestive system a long time, and can help with weight loss because resistant starch acts as a food for your bacteria. This is why only cold potatoes (such as in potato salads), rather than hot ones, are suggested throughout *The Gut Makeover*. The trick is to not let the potatoes dominate your plate so it becomes too beige. I always think the Western industrialised diet looks very beige. Variety is key to the success of *The Gut Makeover*, so try to create a bright, multi-coloured diverse plate at every meal.

Introduce probiotic foods to boost gut flora

Probiotic foods are those which contain live bacteria. In the first fortnight of the plan, dairy foods are left out of the diet to give your gut a chance to repair itself. A damaged gut can find that some proteins in dairy products may trigger inflammation. However, during the reinoculation stage we can add back in some specific dairy products which contain live bacteria that have jobs to do.

I suggest starting on day 14 with a little fermented milk called kefir (see the next page) and also a small crumble of Roquefort cheese and seeing if these sit well with you.

Not having had dairy for a fortnight by this time, it's good to take note of any digestive symptoms. If all is OK, have a bit more kefir the next day, or Roquefort. You could also use other types of fermented foods to boost your bacteria – sauerkraut or pickled fermented vegetables may do the trick.

I am very prescriptive about the type of dairy you put in at this stage, if you can tolerate them. I've chosen the French cheese Roquefort, of all the bacteria-laden cheeses in the supermarket, as it has to be fermented over several weeks in a cave, so when you see the name Roquefort you know it is not a fast-produced cheese and is likely to have a high bacteria count. The reason I suggest kefir, rather than plain yoghurt, is again because it is known to have a very high bacteria count.

Kefir fermented milk

Kefir and fermented milks are used in traditional cooking in many parts of the world. It is a staple of the diet in much of Eastern Europe, and you can find it in most Eastern European corner-shop grocery stores around the UK, and currently online from Tesco and at many of their larger stores in areas where Eastern Europeans live. This means you shouldn't have to go on an expedition to an independent specialist health food store to find it – though you will find the best high-quality organic versions there. If you want to access organic versions easily, they are deliverable from companies like Abel & Cole and Riverford. With the science shining a spotlight on our gut flora and foods which may boost the beneficial strains in your digestive system, it is only a matter of time before kefir becomes a staple of the British diet, too.

The reason I favour kefir above the usual big-brand bacterial strain drinks in supermarkets is because, firstly, it usually does not contain sugar (or artificial sweeteners), and, secondly, the bacterial count in kefir, due to the way it is made, means numbers of bacteria are usually into the double figures of billions. Quality methods of cultivating kefir using living grains and good refrigeration are important in keeping bacterial numbers and variety of species high. The bacteria have to get past the stomach acid and survive into your intestines; many will get killed off on the way, so it's really a numbers game. The more friendly bacteria in the kefir the better, and the more chance the stragglers have of getting through to your lower gut, where they can bloom away.

Kefir also tastes good – once you get used to the texture in your mouth; it's a bit like fizzy milk! You can whizz berries

and other fruits into it, and it becomes a delicious drink. Add
a banana to the mix and you're laughing; the banana contains
prebiotic fibres which the probiotic bacteria from the kefir can
have a feeding frenzy on.

Distinguishing probiotic foods

Companies are no longer allowed to put the word 'probiotic'
on foods, as it is seen as suggesting a health claim. But you
can see some labels reference certain bacterial strains (e.g.
lactobacillus, bifidobacterium or 'live strains'). Sadly, bacterial
counts (how many billions of them) are not shown.

Roquefort cheese

This French cheese is particularly smelly and is fermented for a
long time to create lots of bacteria, which your gut may love. It
is delicious crumbled into salads or as a topping.

Try to get the real Roquefort, not cheap copies, for its full
impact. Do portion-control the cheese, though – a matchbox-size
portion should be the maximum at one meal. Portion-controlled
fat is OK; we need some saturated fat (fats which are hard at
room temperatures) to make cholesterol in the body – this is
needed to make sex hormones and protect our brain. However,
as mentioned on page 43, high-fat diets have been linked with
an unhealthy microbiome, so you should always portion-control
saturated fats, or any fat for that matter.

If you are lactose intolerant

If you cannot tolerate dairy, add live fermented miso to your cooking every day for the last two weeks of this plan. Fermented miso is sold at Asian grocery stores around the UK, and organic versions are sold in independent health food stores. Buy it refrigerated and keep it refrigerated.

Other foods to reintroduce or add

Butter (or organic ghee)

This is also the point when you could start using butter again in your cooking, especially if you find you are tolerating milk dairy products. Butter tastes good, and also comes with a fatty acid called butyrate, which helps build a healthy gut lining, so it can carry on some of the good work you have done in the first fortnight.

If you have problems digesting dairy, try using organic ghee instead of butter for cooking. Ghee contains just 1 per cent lactose and minuscule traces of the protein casein, so many who are lactose intolerant or can't digest casein can still often benefit from it without problems. Ghee contains butyrate, to strengthen the gut lining too.

Fermented tempeh

If you're vegetarian, this is a good protein addition at the halfway point of the plan.

In *The Gut Makeover*, usual supermarket highly-processed tofus and processed soya foods are left out as they can irritate the gut lining. However, fermented soya, such as tempeh, is a type of soya which can be beneficial to the gut. These fermented soyas are thought to be key to better women's hormonal health in Asia. You can buy fermented tempeh in blocks from independent health food stores and Asian supermarkets. You can add it to stir-fries and salads. A recipe is included on page 161. You can also start adding into your diet at this stage some pulses for protein if you are vegetarian. See page 130.

CASE STUDY

Mae

Age: 48

Occupation: Home Maker

Weight before: 14 stone 2lb (89.9kg)

Weight after: 13 stone 3lb (84kg)

Goals: I had stage-three ovarian cancer earlier this year and underwent a major operation, which involved lots of antibiotics straight afterwards. I then had chemotherapy for several months. I suspected this meant my gut flora needed help.

Notes: In the first two weeks, I found the thought of eating 30 varieties of vegetables and fruit daunting. I made an effort to get my vegetable count up at breakfast so I would do scrambled eggs with spinach, tomatoes, ginger, onions and garam masala. Once I was used to it, it was OK. I used to buy the same sort of groceries every week, but this made me look at variety and try new things – for instance I had never tried pak choi or kefir before. I tweaked some of my usual recipes.

I was surprised I was not hungry between meals and I did not get cravings. I used my pressure cooker a lot and had cheaper cuts of organic meat, such as braising steak or neck of lamb, that I cooked till it was tender then added vegetables on top at the end. I made bolognaise with courgette 'spaghetti' and grated parsnips and carrots in to get my vegetable count up; the kids were happy to eat it too.

Eating out was fine – most restaurants can make a big salad and bring you some balsamic vinegar and olive oil to go on top along with some grilled meat or fish. I went to a Brazilian restaurant and they made me a big pile of stir-fried greens with garlic and roasted nuts, and some skewers of meat from the barbecue.

The shakes were really helpful to do in a hurry. I added lots of extras to my kefir in the second half of the plan, such as spinach and berries and pineapple. I used coriander, parsley and rosemary from the garden and added extra herbs to my cooking whenever I could to get the variety of plants up. I boiled ginger and added fresh mint and lemon to it and drank that as a fresh tea. I also made chicken stock using organic chicken carcasses I bought in bulk from the butcher.

Going forward I intend to continue the same eating pattern – especially eating seven-a-day and 30 varieties of plants a week. Overall I feel much better in myself and losing weight is a bonus.

Benefits: My energy levels are massively better, as is my digestion, and my skin is less dry. My menopausal symptoms have also reduced dramatically. Before I had hot flushes every day; now I have just one or two a week. I also lost almost 1 stone (6 kg).

Biggest tip: Clear the house of sweets and temptations before you start.

Summary: What to eat in weeks three and four

Follow the plan from weeks one and two, but add in the following:

- Prebiotic vegetables and fruit – step these up daily. If you want to keep it easy, just remember to have a banana every day. If you want to get more excitement, focus on getting more garlic, onions, leeks, asparagus, Jerusalem artichokes, apples, fennel, cold potatoes and pak choi into your diet. Don't go mad on the cold potatoes – only have a maximum of one-third of your plate. Step up these foods gradually, so your gut can get used to them and to avoid wind issues!
- Probiotic fermented foods – introduce fermented milk kefir and/or fermented miso daily, and introduce small portion-

controlled amounts of smelly fermented Roquefort to your salads or cooking.

- Fats – add butter or ghee to your cooking, in addition to extra virgin olive oil and coconut oil.
- Fermented tempeh – use this if you are vegetarian for extra protein.

The more beneficial bacteria in your gut, the better chance for your weight, immune system, mood and skin. Prebiotic and probiotic foods are worth including in your diet year-round if you can, as they have been shown to reduce the risk of catching colds.

What are you going to eat?

Now you've read the main principles and habits to get used to in *The Gut Makeover*, I'd like to share with you some ideas for ingredients to include in your cooking during this month. Participants of *The Gut Makeover* report really enjoying their food during these weeks and looking forward to all the wonderful, vibrant and filling meals at each main meal.

The key principle is to try to buy food which is as close to its original state as possible and not mucked about with. This is why I recommend shying away, for instance, from almond milk containing 'soya lecithin' (which can, incidentally, irritate the gut lining), or processed meats or sausages containing preservatives and additives. Ask yourself if an ingredient sounds like a food, or a food-like substance? Look for short ingredients lists in foods when shopping, and, if you see something you can't identify as food, and wouldn't use yourself in cooking, leave it.

The following food lists are suggestions of the main foods to incorporate into your diet during your gut makeover, and to give you ideas when planning meals. These lists are designed to fill the core of your shopping lists and to use when stocking your store cupboard and freezer (if you have one).

Foods listed in these categories are a starting point, but feel free to expand the range of quality protein and vegetables if you are more adventurous, or have better access to them. If you think of a meat, fish, seafood, egg or plant not on here, do explore them if you fancy them. However, you should stick with the suggestions for probiotic foods and oils as these are very specific to this programme.

Just remember that whatever you eat or drink needs to be natural and unprocessed to qualify for *The Gut Makeover*.

Meat, fish, seafood and eggs

Meat

- Beef
- Buffalo
- Chicken
- Duck
- Lamb
- Pork
- Turkey
- Organic chicken livers
- Organic calf's liver
- Kidneys
- Ox heart

Game

- Boar
- Grouse
- Pheasant
- Quail
- Rabbit
- Venison

Fish and shellfish

- Anchovies
- Cod
- Crab
- Haddock
- Herring
- Mackerel
- Mussels

- Oysters
- Prawns
- Salmon
- Sardines
- Scallops
- Trout
- Tuna

Eggs

From hens, ducks or quails

Chicken stock

I've included a recipe for how to make real chicken stock on page 171, and I suggest you spoon it into your cooking – from soups and stews to stir-fries – at every opportunity for the collagen to support a strong gut lining.

Shy away from commercial chicken stock cubes if you can – they often contain artificial flavour enhancers and sometimes gluten – or highly processed forms of soya. However, if you haven't time to make your own stock and need something from the supermarket, real chicken stock is now available in the fridge section.

Fats and oils

The following are my preferred choices of fats and oils for *The Gut Makeover*. As you will see, there are no margarine-style spreads (because they are processed foods), or sunflower or vegetable oils (which usually contain higher levels of pro-inflammatory omega-6 fats). The fats and oils in this section have been chosen because they either contain substances shown to be good for the gut, or have anti-inflammatory properties.

- Extra virgin olive oil (mechanical or cold pressed) – make this your main cooking oil and salad oil
- Coconut oil
- Butter or ghee – in the second half of the month

Drinks

- Water – preferably filtered tap water
- Herbal teas, such as fresh ginger steeped in boiling water
- Unsweetened almond milk
- Coconut water
- Chicory root. This makes a good coffee replacement. It contains inulin, which is a prebiotic to boost beneficial bacteria in the gut. It can be mixed with warmed unsweetened almond milk for a latte substitute, but take care to limit to one a day due to its potential laxative effect. Buy the 100 per cent organic chicory roasted powder if you can – beware of liquid versions which are mixed with sugar.

Nuts and seeds

These will be used principally in cooking. Nuts and seeds are highly nutritious and filled with minerals and vitamins. They also contain protein and fibre to fill you up, and the oils carry many health benefits too. Many nuts contain zinc, which is necessary for a healthy gut lining.

So nuts and seeds can be beneficial, but you need to be careful on portions as high-fat diets have been linked with an unfavourable microbiome (as mentioned on page 43). Here are some ideas of nuts and seeds to include in your meals:

- Almonds
- Brazil nuts
- Cashews
- Chestnuts
- Hazelnuts
- Macadamias
- Peanuts
- Pecans
- Pine nuts
- Pistachios
- Pumpkin seeds
- Sesame seeds (black or gold)
- Sunflower seeds
- Walnuts

Vegetables

Those marked in bold below are prebiotic gut flora boosters. You may need to introduce them slowly into your diet, as initially they can cause wind, but this should lessen as your gut flora becomes more balanced.

- **Asparagus**
- Aubergines
- Beetroot
- Broccoli
- Brussels sprouts
- Cabbage
- Carrots
- Cauliflower
- Celeriac
- Celery
- Chard
- **Chicory root**
- **Cold potatoes**
- Courgettes

- Cucumbers
- **Fennel**
- Garlic
- Green beans
- **Jerusalem artichokes**
- Kale
- **Leeks**
- Lettuce
- Mushrooms
- Okra (ladies' fingers)
- **Onions**
- Peas
- **Pak choi**
- Parsnips

- Peppers (capsicum)
- Pumpkin
- Radicchio
- Radishes
- Rocket
- Romanesco
- Spinach
- Squash
- Swede
- Sweet potatoes
- Sweetcorn
- Tomatoes
- Watercress

Tips

- Both **onions** and **garlic** are more powerful prebiotics when raw. You can eat red onions or white, but the red pigment is a bonus as it contains anti-inflammatory plant chemical anthocyanins.
- **Squash**, **pumpkin** and **sweet potatoes** can be bought ready peeled and chopped in supermarkets nowadays. If freshly peeled and chopped yourself, they contain more nutrients than ready-chopped, but if the time and awkwardness of dissecting a squash yourself is the difference between you eating it or not eating it, buy ready-chopped. The vitamin A in the orange pigments is a great nutrient for building your gut lining.

Herbs, spices and condiments

These have the potential to make this plan doable or not doable
– and save you from boredom by introducing different flavours
and textures to your everyday diet. Many herbs are anti-
inflammatory, as well as providing diversity for the microbiome,
so snip them up and liberally use them in your cooking as much
as you can. They are not all about just taste.

- Basil
- Bay leaves
- Black pepper
- Cayenne pepper
- Coriander
- Cumin
- Dill
- Dried red chillies
- Fish sauce
- **Garlic**
- Ginger
- Kalamata olives
- Mint
- Mustard
- Pomegranate molasses
- Preserved or pickled lemons
- Rosemary
- Saffron
- Sea salt
- Sichuan peppers
- Sumac
- Tamari soy sauce
- Tarragon
- Thyme
- Turmeric (this is a powerful anti-inflammatory)
- Vinegars – including balsamic, red wine vinegar and apple cider vinegar

Tips

- **Kalamata olives** are usually a purple colour. Do not eat the dark black olives which have been dyed – we want to keep your diet unprocessed.

- **Mustard** comes in a number of varieties. Go for French, not English, as English often contains gluten – though the powdered version doesn't.
- **Sea salt** contains minerals. I like Ibiza salt or Maldon.
- **Sichuan peppers (also known as Szechuan peppercorns or Sichuan flower chilli peppers)** are now stocked by some supermarkets, or you can get them online or from an Asian grocery store. They are worth the effort; they have a lovely lemony, peppery flavour.
- **Sumac** is popular in the Middle East and now available in supermarkets. It has a wonderful lime taste rubbed into meats and fish.
- **Tamari sauce** is gluten-free, unlike soy sauce.
- **Vinegars,** such as balsamic, red wine vinegar and apple cider vinegar, can be used in dressings or on salads.

Fruits

- **Apples**
- Apricots (*fresh* not dried)
- Avocados
- **Bananas**
- Blackberries
- Blackcurrants
- Blueberries
- Cherries
- Clementines
- Figs
- Gooseberries
- Grapefruit
- Grapes
- Kiwis
- Lemons
- Limes
- Mangoes
- Melons
- Mulberries
- Nectarines
- Oranges
- Papayas

- Passion Fruits
- Peaches
- Pears
- Pineapples
- Plums
- Pomegranates
- Quinces
- Raspberries
- Rhubarb
- Satsumas
- Strawberries
- Tangerines
- Watermelon

Prebiotic foods

I've highlighted the prebiotic foods in the above lists using bold text, but here is a complete list of the approved prebiotic foods.

- Apples
- Asparagus
- Bananas
- Chicory root
- Cold potatoes (not hot!)
- Fennel
- Garlic
- Jerusalem artichokes
- Leeks
- Onions
- Pak choi
- Pulses (only allowed if you are vegetarian on the second half of the makeover to boost sources of protein)

Probiotic foods

- Kefir fermented milk
- Roquefort
- Fermented live miso – available in the fridge section of Asian supermarkets and many independent health food stores
- Fermented tempeh – available in the fridge section of Asian supermarkets and health food stores

Hannah

Age: 38

Occupation: PR director

Weight before: 12 stone (76.2kg)

Weight after: 11 stone 5lb (72kg)

Goals: I wanted to lose weight, sleep better and improve my skin quality.

Notes: In the first three to four days I felt quite sluggish and had headaches, even though I had reduced my caffeine intake slowly in the preceding week. I had been on five cups of tea a day, then reduced to two a day in the week before the make-over, then came off it altogether when I started the plan.

I had been worried that I would feel hungry but actually I didn't until right before a mealtime. I ate two pieces of fruit a day so that gave me the sweetness I needed.

I really enjoyed thinking about what I was cooking; that is something I have come away with. It is interesting to look for new recipes and cook new things. I have substituted the pasta and grains easily with cauliflower rice and courgettes in the shape of pasta, and used sweet potatoes with meals.

Don't assume this plan will be expensive. I was making my own lunch every day so it was not more expensive.

I have picked up some good habits, such as automatically going for vegetables to get my count up each day, and having as many different types as possible with every meal.

My alcohol tolerance is now lower and I feel strongly about not having it on an empty stomach. If I am going out for drinks I make sure I eat before or with it, drink slower and have some non-alcoholic drinks too. I know that keeping the alcohol low is a big thing for my weight.

Benefits: I lost half a stone (3kg) and 11cm (4in) came off my waist. My sleep is much better. People say my skin looks brighter and better, but it is hard to say, because I was on medication for adult acne (not an antibiotic by the way!) for nine months which stopped at the same time I came to the end of the makeover. I used to wake at 4am a lot but in the four weeks of the makeover this hardly happened at all. That made a difference. I had terrible anxiety before and that has subsided. I have to confess, I'm amazed at the results.

Biggest tip: If you are out and about, a good safety option is a Niçoise salad; these are widely sold nowadays.

The cost of eating well

There can be a worry that eating for health is expensive. However, with planning and focus, it does not have to be this way. In this plan there are mainly piles of vegetables and some protein, cooked deliciously.

Organic vegetables and fruit are great if you can afford them – to benefit from the lack of pesticides and the lower toxic burden – however you can still do this plan using regular well-washed ones. Vegetables can be picked up cheaply – at the grocery stores on street corners selling a bowl for a pound and discount supermarkets, for starters. As long as you wash non-organic vegetables and fruits thoroughly, you can enjoy the colours and fibre to enhance your microbiome.

For wild fish at cheap prices, look in the freezer section of your supermarket. You can buy bags of frozen fillets of haddock, cod and mackerel, which are all wild and antibiotic-free, in major stores – often working out less than 80p per fillet. Wild Alaskan salmon can be bought, frozen, in many supermarkets for £1 a fillet. Just remember to take it out of the freezer on the morning you want to cook it. Smoked mackerel fillets with peppercorns often work out at £1 a fillet and make a quick lunch protein. Tinned fish is also an inexpensive healthy protein. For example, tinned sardines in olive oil make an easy lunch protein and, again, are wild. Eating the soft bones in them will give you a shot of calcium at cheap prices – a tin can be as little as 40p.

Organ meats are fantastic sources of nutrients – packing in more vitamins and minerals per square centimetre than regular flesh. If you venture into this area, it is probably best to go organic to minimise the antibiotic load. The liver is the processing plant of an animal, and if antibiotics have been administered, this is the most likely organ to retain residues. You can get three meals out of a packet of organic chicken livers sold for less than £3.

Organic eggs may cost double the price of regular ones, but they are a relatively cost-effective source of protein, often working out about 50p per egg. Organic chicken, if bought in fillets, can be prohibitively expensive (for example, in my local supermarket chicken breasts cost £20 a kilogram), but if you buy a whole organic chicken, you can get several meals out of one. For instance, you could buy a medium-sized organic chicken in super-markets for around £11. On the first night you can roast it. You could then pick the remaining meat off it for another day and boil the bones to make a large jar of gelatinous and nutritious stock, which you can keep in the fridge for several days to add to soups and stir-fries. The day after roasting the chicken, you could use picked cold chicken in a salad for dinner. And the next day you could have a stir-fry with the remaining meat. So an £11 organic chicken could provide the protein for multiple meals, plus at least 1kg (2lb) of chicken stock to boost the nutrient content (micro minerals and collagen) for several soups and other meals after-wards. A kilogram of chicken stock in a supermarket might cost you £6 alone, and probably wouldn't even be organic, so making your own is a cost-effective as well as healthy option.

Another strategy for picking up organic meat and fish at a fraction of the normal price is to head to your local supermarket at the time of day when the big, final-hour reductions take place just before the sell-by date runs out. Often 5pm is the appointed hour, but you may need to pop in a few times or ask other locals who are in the know what is the magic time. If you can load up with reduced foods that are still perfectly safe and nutritious to eat, you could then bung a pile of organic produce in the freezer till needed.

Remember, junk food isn't always cheap either. For the same price as a big brand pizza you could treat yourself to a good-quality organic steak for dinner or a packet of wild Alaskan smoked salmon which would cover your protein needs for a couple of meals.

In some of the breakfast recipes I have suggested using chia seeds or flaxseeds. If you're on a budget flaxseeds are usually the cheaper option. Chia and flax are both full of omega-3 essential fatty acids, which are anti-inflammatory and may support gut health. They draw water into them and swell up in your intestines, which triggers contractions to keep everything moving along and avoid constipation. Flaxseeds are also called linseeds, and can be bought ready ground, or in seed form, in high street supermarkets and health food shops.

I suggest stocking up on nuts and seeds cheaply in bulk from the discount retailers before you start this plan – as they work out cheaper than the small packets from supermarkets. Once opened, put a clip on the packet to make it airtight and store in the door of your fridge. Nuts and seeds, once opened, can go rancid if left exposed to air or kept in warm places.

Berries, such as blueberries and raspberries, can be bought more economically frozen. As they are frozen immediately after being picked they retain decent quantities of vitamins and minerals and, of course, fibre. When frozen, they are ideal for whizzing in a shake in the morning as, being cold, they can make the drink feel refreshing.

The Gut Makeover is alcohol- and caffeine-free, so you may save money there. Add up what you normally spend in a month on bottles of wine at home, plus any lattes, macchiatos and alcoholic drinks when you're out, and see how much this gives you to invest in better-quality foods for a month.

CASE STUDY

Peter

Age: 53

Occupation: Lawyer

Weight before: 14 stone 1lb (89.2kg)

Weight after: 13 stone 6lb (85.1kg)

Goals: To get healthy. It would also be good to lose some weight.

Notes: I wanted to be healthier. I wanted to look after myself better. My uncle died of stomach cancer. Before *The Gut Makeover*, sometimes when things got going, four glasses of wine would go down very fast. I was having a whole pot of black tea in the morning and I was stuck in a bad habit of snacking at 11am and 4pm on dark chocolate. At lunchtime, I would have two large slices of bread with processed meats and a piece of fruit, usually 'al desko', and I would wolf it down. It didn't feel good, but I was doing it.

When my wife and I started *The Gut Makeover* it was also a chance for me to get more involved in the cooking. I used to, but that had fallen off. Initially it felt a big challenge. At first, you think of the things you cannot eat, but quickly the recipes meant the diet felt good. When you are faced with tasty, filling protein and a big plateful of vegetables or salad, you find yourself asking: how am I going to lose weight eating all this?

We went to the supermarket and spent a lot of time in the vegetable section. There were whole aisles of the supermarket we didn't go into any more – dairy, processed meats, crisps, alcohol. A big change of routine, but no big deal, once you have another direction.

The core of *The Gut Makeover* is wonderful things you can enjoy and you don't feel at all deprived once you get going. I have had no cravings mid-morning or afternoon.

Longer term, I'm not going back to caffeine. I feel less on edge and more cool and collected without it. I'm going to drink alcohol in a different way: I am going to have a drink when I think, 'Ooh, that would be nice.' Not just routinely slosh it down. I don't want to load that onto my system any more.

Benefits: I lost 9lb (4kg) in weight. I had to go to Gap and buy new jeans in a size down – the first time in ten years! My violent sneezing after eating has also gone and I'm enjoying cooking.

Biggest tip: It is good to do *The Gut Makeover* with someone; for example, with your partner or a friend. There is a lot of new stuff and you can encourage each other.

Strategies for success

If you don't normally cook from scratch, you may find this plan mildly challenging at first, but once you're in a rhythm, have written your shopping lists, tried new recipes, packed your freezer, used your blender and perhaps started eating leftovers for lunch out of a plastic pot (not at your desk!) or found alternative items to sandwiches in the canteen or local lunch shops, habits will form and become part of your new routine.

The key to a successful *Gut Makeover* is the planning. If you go out unprepared, or without visualising what the next meal will be, you may fall at the first hurdle. If it's late and you haven't got any *Gut Makeover* meals planned or defrosted, you may end up making poor food choices out of hunger and find yourself back where you started with your health.

At work, try to get into the habit of having fresh food with you in a box or a piece of fruit, and warn colleagues that you are eating your own food when the ciabattas are trollied into meetings.

The next suggestion is really a last resort, but have you thought about long-life foods you could have if stuck? Perhaps you could stash a jar of artichokes in olive oil, a tin of sardines, a tin or jar of olives, an apple and a bottle of coconut water in your desk drawer or car boot. You probably have ideas of your own you could store for an emergency meal. I'm not suggesting this is the way to eat every day, but if you find it's this or a late-night takeaway pizza, or stopping by a petrol station on the way home from work and having a Pot Noodle, then you have your secret supports to help you keep on track. Plan to succeed!

You don't need to hibernate for a month and miss parties with this plan; you just need a strategy for social events. I've had various periods of abstinence and, to dodge the 'you're so boring' taunts, I don't advertise I'm on the wagon. Have you noticed how friends will congratulate you if you pause drinking for charity for a month but if you do it for your health – well, that's another matter? I usually profess thirst on arrival and ask for a glass of water, and then after that nobody notices that I'm drinking sparkling water with a slice of lime.

Nowadays it's easy to check menus online before eating out, which means you can think about what you are going to order before you get to a restaurant. If the menu looks unable to cater for your protein/plant plan, you could always ring ahead and ask. Many places will happily sauté a nice steak, or cook a piece of fish and produce a large salad or pile of crispy vegetables for you.

All restaurants in the EU now have to be able to explain what foods on their menu contain allergens, so finding out about use of dairy and gluten is much easier. Chain restaurants are particularly well prepared for these questions – you often get handed a whole table of information.

If you know you struggle with willpower, think about asking a buddy to do *The Gut Makeover* with you. Doing it with your other half, flatmate, friend, colleague or neighbour can make the journey more fun, and can increase your chances of success as you can support each other along the way. On a practical level, you may even be able to save time by cooking in batches and swapping some of the portions with your buddy or neighbour without having to make two different meals. You can also swap recipes and ideas.

If you need more help to keep on track, like the *Gut Makeover* Facebook page. This online support group can be invaluable for sharing strategies and recipes and chatting to others with similar goals.

CASE STUDY

Marion

Age: 57

Occupation: Creative producer

Weight before: 10 stone 8lb (67kg)

Weight after: 10 stone 1lb (64kg)

Goals: To get healthier and lose a bit of weight. I have irritable bowel syndrome and I wanted to see if *The Gut Makeover* would help my digestive system to work better.

Notes: Before *The Gut Makeover* I used to drink three glasses of wine every evening. I had the habit of drinking while cooking the evening meal. The wine: it is a funny thing – it's pretty much in the head. Once I started *The Gut Makeover*, the wine became secondary because I became so focused on the diet and doing something good for my health. I was not just eating for the sake of eating; I was nourishing myself.

The biggest challenge for me was the planning and getting organised. I photocopied the meal plans from the book and the list of foods to eat, and stuck them on the kitchen wall. I used a lot of recipes from the book, and also adapted some of my own.

I did the plan with my husband, and I was asking on the Facebook private group about portion sizes near the beginning as we were eating a lot. We were eating more than before, but in fact, both of us lost weight.

My IBS has now gone – it's the first time I have not been suffering with loose stools since I was 15 years old! I feel inclined to carry on with this style of eating longer term. I will go back to wine, but at the weekend – definitely not every day – and will have it as a treat. I am going to try some sourdough bread and see if gluten triggers my IBS symptoms again. If it does, I will consider cutting it out long term.

The Gut Makeover was a revelation for us. We have really enjoyed it.

Benefits: This was my first respite from IBS in 42 years and I lost 7lb (3kg). I was in Paris for the last three days of the plan and all my friends told me that I looked different – really healthy and great.

Biggest tip: Try to get organised the week before you start. Prepare some of the new things such as boiled potatoes to keep in the fridge and make the banana bread. Start the week with a roast chicken because then you have a base for meals for the next three days sorted.

Frequently asked questions

The *Gut Makeover* Facebook page (www.facebook.com/TheGutMakeover) is our online community to get advice, ask questions and share tips and success stories, but I have included some of the most frequently asked questions here. Do come and join us online!

Are cold potatoes counted in my plant portions each day?

We all know they are a vegetable and one that I have recommended for this plan (see page 61), but I suggest not counting them in your seven a day, to encourage you to use the count for more brightly coloured plants and focus on expanding your range.

Can I drink decaffeinated coffee or tea?

Many decaffeinated drinks have gone through extra processing to take the caffeine out and still usually contain a small amount of caffeine. The aim of *The Gut Makeover* is to fill your body with unprocessed natural foods and drinks, so for this month it would be better to find other options; rooibos (also called redbush) tea is a good replacement for black tea, or try ground chicory with unsweetened almond milk instead of a coffee. See page 74 for other ideas. Some *Gut Makeover* participants have said it was easier and more enjoyable to adopt completely new drinks instead. I've noticed herbal tea selections have come a long way since the days of just fruit teas or peppermint, and there are some pretty decent blends on the market now.

You mention bitter salads and pineapple as starters. Can I just make a bigger bitter salad with pineapple and call it a main meal instead?

I've suggested introducing starter salads and plants when you can. This is not just for the digestive support but because it's another really convenient way of getting in another vegetable portion in an enjoyable way. Also, making a starter on a weekday, when many of us may not normally think about it, can make a meal feel a bit more special in minutes. But, yes, you can always double the quantity and add a portion of protein on the side, such as a tin of fish or some smoked flaked salmon, to make it into a main meal.

What should I do if I don't want to lose weight on *The Gut Makeover*, but I want to follow it for all the other health benefits that can come with it?

- Don't implement the 12-hour overnight fast.
- Have a mid-afternoon snack of nuts and fruit between lunch and dinner.

- Be more liberal with your oils and fats in cooking and include more fatty foods in the plan, such as nuts and seeds, avocados and coconut milk, and in the second fortnight be more generous with the Roquefort and the butter.

I've noticed after the first week I don't feel particularly hungry even several hours after breakfast. Should I still try to eat protein with lunch, even if I just fancy a vegetable soup or a light pile of salad?

In the first week of the plan it's important to have protein with every meal as this anchors your blood sugar levels and makes you feel full up for many hours. This means higher chances of this plan being a success, as there is less opportunity of falling into a state of ravenous hunger and making poor food choices.

Many of those who have already done *The Gut Makeover* say that after one week of diligently eating protein with each meal, while cutting out sugar and grains, their hunger levels plummet, and some say that, to their surprise, they don't have much appetite at all. If this happens, adjust your portions sizes to your reduced appetite. You could reduce the meat or fish at one of your daily meals – for instance, make lunch or dinner a soup or light salad with just a few nuts or seeds sprinkled on top.

I'm vegetarian – can I still do *The Gut Makeover*?

Absolutely! *The Gut Makeover* is based on hunter-gatherers' diets as these people have the most enviable microbiomes and consequently largely avoid the non-communicable diseases ravaging the Western world, such as obesity, diabetes, heart disease and cancer. Their reliance on a massive range of different plants is most likely a big factor.

Eating a massive variety of vegetables and fruits on *The Gut Makeover* can support a healthy gut and could be a good way to improve your health if you are vegetarian and not reaching these levels already. The core *Gut Makeover* programme doesn't include pulses – including chickpeas, lentils, red kidney beans, etc. – nor the type of highly processed soya or mycoprotein Quorn found in regular supermarkets. In the first fortnight you can have eggs, nuts and seeds for protein. However, in the second fortnight (the 'Reinoculate' phase), you will add in butter to your cooking to keep the repair going and introduce bacteria from kefir fermented milk and Roquefort cheese, which both contain protein, so these could be enjoyed too if you are vegetarian. In this Reinoculate stage you could also introduce some fermented soya, such as tempeh (see page 103). I have included a recipe using tempeh on page 161.

If you are vegetarian, you can also start adding pulses back into your diet in the second half of the programme (weeks three and four) so that you have additional sources of protein. If you do this, introduce them bit by bit to avoid bloating: starting with a spoonful of hummus and add a little more the next day. Add them to soups and casseroles where the pulses will be well cooked so that they are easier to digest.

Sara (vegetarian)

Age: 31

Occupation: PR

Weight before: 8 stone 9lb (54.9kg)

Weight after: 8 stone (50.8kg)

Goals: To get rid of bloating.

Notes: I have never done a 'diet' before. I was attracted by the fact there is such a health benefit to this programme.

For years, I felt like a lot of things were irritating my stomach. I didn't realise how badly till I did *The Gut Makeover.* I thought my digestive problems weren't extreme, but I was living with discomfort. I used to get bloating every day, and I sometimes looked six months' pregnant. I also suffered from migraines.

I felt better as soon as I started *The Gut Makeover.* I didn't suffer withdrawal headaches from caffeine, because I don't drink it. I immediately noticed the bloating went and I felt less sluggish. I also stopped having afternoon dips when I'd reach for biscuits and then need a big bowl of pasta for dinner when I got home. That emotional response to food went straight away. It feels life-changing how much more comfortable I feel and it has been lovely to lose a few pounds in weight too.

As a vegetarian, there were less protein options for me to eat in the first two weeks, so I focused on nuts and seeds plus eggs. For breakfast I had onion, garlic, chillies, lime and spinach with a couple of eggs cracked in the middle, which kept me going all morning. I had a handful of almonds or other nuts or seeds in my evening meals for the protein there. In the second half of the plan I used fermented soya tempeh for protein as well. Even though we could add kefir and Roquefort cheese for protein in the second half, I didn't as I have an aversion to dairy and don't like it. I did add in some pulses; I tried some lentils in moderate amounts in soups, and I did try black beans one evening in a Mexican dish with guacamole, but it gave me bloating again, so I stopped that.

At the end of the plan, I may gradually increase pulses in my diet, but then introduce them very gradually and monitor my symptoms to identify which ones may not agree with me. I can then tweak my diet accordingly. I am wondering if cutting out gluten has been a big help, and will reintroduce that over a few days to check if that is a trigger.

Benefits: I have dropped a dress size, my chronic bloating has disappeared and I no longer have migraines.

Biggest tip: When you're strict about having a good lunch and good dinner, the cravings just go.

What advice do you have for shopping and navigating the supermarket?

The shorter the ingredients list the better. If you don't under-stand it, don't buy it. This plan is focused on natural food. I like to look at ingredients lists on the sides of food in supermarkets and think, 'If I was making that myself would I put it in there?' Freezing is a good way to preserve food without having to add anything man-made or artificial to it.

Are nuts and seeds counted in our 20–30 varieties of plants each week?

Although, of course, these are plants, I suggest not including them in the plant count as they are high in fat and the more we can focus on the bright colours and fibre filling the plate, the better. The vegetable side of our diet is the bit most of us need the spotlight on.

Is it OK to use frozen vegetables or fruit?

Yes! These foods contain lots of fibre, and are usually frozen soon after picking and so retain many of their nutrients. Frozen peas or sweetcorn can provide a nice quick portion of your seven a day. Frozen berries are cheaper than fresh ones, and are great blended into a shake from frozen.

What if I'm having a hectic week at work so have to grab food on the go?

Breakfast: Buy everything you need for your morning shakes and store. Unsweetened almond milk or kefir usually have longish use-by dates, so you can have those in the fridge ready. You could buy frozen fruit to go in the shake, to also save time on chopping, cutting, or risking them going off between your weekly shops, if that is the way you shop. Add nuts and/or seeds to the shake for the protein and healthy fats to make you feel full for a few hours.

Lunch: Admittedly, sandwich and convenience shops are often full of beige food – pasties, sandwiches, crisps and fizzy drinks – but many of the larger chains are cottoning on to the fact that people want to eat fresh and healthy produce. You can usually get a fresh fruit salad in M&S or Pret, for example. Head to the non-sandwich end of the store – get a pack of olives, roasted marinated peppers and perhaps a small pack of cooked, roast, sliced chicken or flaked salmon. Buy some coconut water.

Dinner: For evening meals at home, cook ahead – your freezer is going to be the font of good meals – but if you've run out of those and you have to go to a supermarket, look for protein and plant meals with short ingredients lists (which means fewer processed or artificial ingredients).

Another option is to have a shake for dinner, such as a green shake, which gets lots of plants and some nuts and seeds protein in there. Then you can open a packet of smoked mackerel or smoked salmon and have that with a couple of chopped, ready-baked beetroots from the supermarket.

If you're heading out in the evening, think about eating before you get there – then there's less chance of getting into a state of severe hunger and making poor food choices just because cheese and wine is all that is provided.

If you need to eat out, Nando's is a good bet! Grilled peri-peri chicken for the protein, with a portion of corn on the cob and a portion of green peas in chilli and mint. Their chicken is British sourced and carries the Red Tractor farm assurance endorsement, so for a 'fast food' restaurant, is at the better end of the quality scale. Check with staff there is no gluten in any of the additional chilli sauces you might want to put on top, and out will come their allergens manual.

I had more bloating than usual in the first couple of days of *The Gut Makeover*. Why is this?

You may be eating many more vegetables generally than normal, and the gut can take time to adjust to a new style of eating. In addition, some individuals' guts can be a little sensitive at first to prebiotic foods, such as bananas (see the full list on page 116). If you experience bloating with these, only start building them up in your diet very gradually.

If you are one of the 30 per cent of the population potentially with a sensitivity to gluten, you may find your digestive system takes time to settle down when gluten and other grains you might have been reacting to are taken out of your diet. Constipation and a bit of temporary bloating can result while the gut is getting over the shock of the new. If this happens, build up your plant portions gradually – especially the prebiotic ones – and be sure to keep hydrated with water and herbal teas.

Put two large spoonfuls of flaxseeds (also known as linseeds) or chia seeds into your shake in the morning for a laxative effect if you find you have gone a day without a bowel movement.

Summary

So now you've seen the types of ingredients you'll be using over these four weeks, let's look at some recipes. You can use the ingredients lists on pages 109–116 to create some of your own meals or make a few simple adaptions to any favourite recipes you already have. I also hope the recipes in this book will excite you to try new dishes too.

PART THREE

Recipes and meal plans

Introduction

Now you've read the compelling science behind *The Gut Makeover*, here are the guidelines for the four-week plan to transform your gut health. On *The Gut Makeover* you'll be enjoying three delicious meals a day, teeming with nutrients and with huge variety, without counting calories or going hungry. There are breakfasts that include eggs, banana nut 'breads', 'creamy' nut and fruit shakes, and the odd green smoothie thrown in for good measure. Lunches and dinners include lots of variety, from lamb and Thai curries to potato salads, bolognaises and Niçoise salads, roast chicken with lots of roast veg, meatballs with almonds, roasted peppers drizzled in extra virgin olive oil, warm salads, cooked grated carrots with walnuts and brightly coloured stir-fries, to name a few. Every meal includes mountains of vegetables and some fruits, cooked in delicious and enticing ways using the best of condiments, herbs and spices to keep life interesting and satisfying.

Mouth watering now? Let's begin.

Note: Depending on their ingredients, some of these recipes are designed either for first two weeks of the *Gut Makeover* ('Phase One'), or for the second two weeks ('Phase Two'): others are suited for anytime in the month. All recipes are marked with a ①, a ② or both, to let you know which phase(s) they're best for.

Breakfasts

A liquid breakfast can be very easy and welcome in the morning – particularly when you're not terribly hungry. A breakfast in a glass can slip down more easily than food you have to chew.

GREEN GUNGE ① ②

Serves 2

I'm not going to mince my words – call a green smoothie what you like, but in the end it's basically gunge! It's palatable gunge, of course, and has the advantage of being a practical way to get lots of fibre and a variety of plants down you in one sitting. Here, the almonds are added for protein and good fats, which will keep you feeling full for longer. The ginger and mint are anti-inflammatory. If you can't warm to the taste of a green smoothie but want to give it a go, sipping it through a straw will hide a lot of its flavour; but personally, with the zing of ginger and lime, I like this concoction.

2 cups kale or spinach, washed
1 cup filtered water
1 orange, peeled
50g almonds
3 fresh mint leaves
1 lime, squeezed
2cm fresh ginger, grated

Add all the ingredients to a blender, and blitz.

Tip: If you have time, soaking the almonds overnight in water makes it easier for your blender to break them up and easier for you to digest them.

GREEN SHAKE ① ②

Serves 2

2 handfuls of kale or spinach, washed
1 fennel bulb, chopped
2 ripe kiwis
1 apple
¼ cucumber
1cm fresh ginger, unpeeled
½ lime, peeled
A handful of fresh mint leaves
250ml filtered water

Add all the ingredients to a blender and pulse until smooth. Taste for texture – if you prefer your shake a little less thick, add more water to dilute it.

Drink immediately, before the ingredients separate.

NUTTY NON-DAIRY BREAKFAST SHAKE ① ②

Serves 1

200ml unsweetened almond milk
½ cup frozen berries
½ banana
1 tbsp ground flaxseeds (also called linseeds)

Blend all the ingredients together in a blender until smooth and drink immediately. If left to stand, the shake will become thicker as the flax swells up, and then you'll need to eat it with a spoon.

Follow by drinking a glass of water to aid the digestion of the flax.

KEFIR + PINEAPPLE BREAKFAST SHAKE ②

Serves 1

If you are in a hurry you can use the ready-chopped pineapple that you find in the fridge section of the supermarket.

200ml kefir
1 cup chopped fresh pineapple
2cm fresh ginger, peeled
2 tsp chia seeds or ground flaxseeds

Add all the ingredients to a blender and pulse until smooth. Drink immediately, before the ingredients separate.

Follow by drinking a large glass of water to help the digestion of the chia or flax seeds.

Tip: If you have time, soaking the chia seeds in water overnight makes it easier for your blender to break them up.

KEFIR + BERRIES ②

Serves 1

200ml kefir

1 cup frozen berries

½ banana

2 tsp chia seeds or ground flaxseeds

1cm fresh ginger

Blend all the ingredients together in a blender then drink immediately before the ingredients separate.

Tip: If you have time, soaking the chia seeds in water overnight makes it easier for your blender to break them up.

SPINACH + POTATO SCRAMBLED EGG ① ②

Serves 1

The cold potatoes add a prebiotic to this meal, as they are a resistant starch food. Although you can still get resistant starch from slightly reheated cold new potatoes, this does not give you licence to turn *The Gut Makeover* into a fried chip diet!

1 tbsp extra virgin olive oil

2 small new potatoes, pre-boiled and chilled

A really large handful of spinach, washed

1 large egg, beaten

Sea salt

Heat the oil in a pan over a medium heat. Add the potatoes and sauté gently for a few moments.

Add the spinach to the pan and cook until it has wilted.

Stir the beaten egg into the potatoes and spinach until the egg is set.

Sprinkle with a little sea salt to your taste and serve.

SCRAMBLED EGGS WITH SALMON   ①②

Serves 1

2 slices of wild Alaskan smoked salmon
2 medium eggs, beaten
1 tbsp extra virgin olive oil (phase 1)

or

1 knob of butter or ghee (phase 2)

Cut the slices of salmon into small strips.

Heat the oil or butter in a pan over a medium heat, add the eggs and salmon, and keep stirring, until the egg is set and the salmon has changed colour slightly.

WILD SALMON + AVOCADO   ①②

Serves 1

1 ripe avocado, peeled and sliced
2 slices of wild Alaskan smoked salmon
½ lemon
Freshly ground black pepper

Arrange the avocado and salmon on a plate, squeeze over the lemon juice and season with pepper, to taste.

BANANA NUT BREAKFAST BREAD   ① ②

Makes 1 loaf

Make this at the weekend and have it ready for the mornings over the next week, so you have something delicious to hand when you need to conjure up breakfast quickly. A slice of this is a satisfying accompaniment to one of the shakes if you need more protein in the morning to keep you going. This has been adapted from a recipe by the Nutritional Therapist/Chef Christine Bailey.

2 tbsp extra virgin olive oil
2 cups walnuts
1 cup ground almonds
2 tsp baking powder (gluten-free if available)
1 ripe banana
3 large eggs
2 tbsp honey

Grease a loaf tin with a little of the olive oil. Preheat the oven to 180°C.

Grind the walnuts in a blender. Add the ground walnuts to the ground almonds and baking powder in a mixing bowl.

Put the banana, eggs, remaining olive oil and honey in the blender and mix until all broken down. Add the wet mixture to the dry mixture and stir with a wooden spoon.

Pour the batter into the loaf tin and bake for 30 minutes, or until a skewer comes out of the mixture clean.

Remove from the oven, turn out, and allow to cool.

CHIA CAVIAR   ① ②

This makes a great breakfast served with fresh fruit and scattered with nuts and seeds, but it's equally delicious as a dessert.

240ml unsweetened almond milk or kefir (phase 2)
2 tbsp chia seeds

Mix the ingredients together in a bowl or large glass and place in the fridge.

Every 15 minutes for 2 hours, go back to the fridge and stir the caviar. You should end up with a soft pearl-like consistency, which you can use as a delicious dessert served alongside either a portion of berries or a couple of slices of fresh mango.

Lunches and Dinners

This section gives ideas for making more substantial *Gut Makeover* meals. Some can be knocked up at lunchtime, while others make good evening meals, which in turn can provide delicious leftovers for lunch the next day.

CHICORY + APPLE SALAD ①②

Serves 1

Chicory is a slightly bitter vegetable, so it can stimulate production of your stomach acid to help with digestion. The apples have prebiotic properties to help your gut flora flourish.

2 chicory heads, washed and sliced
1 apple, peeled, cored and sliced
A handful of walnuts, chopped

For the dressing:
Juice of ½ lemon
2 tbsp extra virgin olive oil
1 garlic clove, peeled and finely chopped

Combine all the salad ingredients in a bowl. Mix the dressing ingredients in a glass with a fork and drizzle over the salad.

CHICORY + PINE NUT + ROQUEFORT ②

Serves 2

140g red or green chicory (about 3 small heads), washed and sliced
1 knob butter
50g pine nuts
A sprinkle of dried chilli flakes, to taste (optional)
A sprinkle of sea salt flakes
2 tbsp extra virgin olive oil
Juice of ½ lemon
Matchbox-sized piece of Roquefort

Put the chicory in a bowl.

Melt the butter in a frying pan over a medium heat. Add the pine nuts and sprinkle with the chilli flakes, if using, and sea salt. Move the nuts around the pan to coat them well with the butter and flavourings. Cook until the pine nuts are golden brown. Watch them carefully as they burn easily.

Sprinkle the warm nuts over the chicory and drizzle with the olive oil and lemon juice. Crumble the cheese over, if using.

Serve at once.

MARIO'S ORANGE SALAD   ①②

Serves 2

Our Italian friend Mario invited us to his gorgeous shack on the River Thames in London recently while I was writing this book. He's a brilliant cook – homemade pizzas in his 350°C oven being his speciality. We said we'd love to come, then dropped the gluten-free bombshell. Unfazed, Mario conjured up a superb meal and this was his Italian starter, containing the perfect ingredients to stimulate stomach acid production and help digestion. A perfect example of cultural cooking and the real Mediterranean diet that is so good for the gut. This salad was followed by a baked sea bass each.

Use Kalamata olives as they are not processed and dyed black like some other varieties.

2 large oranges, peeled, halved and sliced into half moons
1 red onion, peeled and thinly sliced into half moons
3 tbsp extra virgin olive oil
2 tbsp Kalamata olives, stoned and chopped
1 small tin of anchovies in olive oil, chopped

Assemble all the ingredients in a salad bowl and serve immediately.

TRIPLE GREENS   ①②

Serves 2

It is important to get as much variety of vegetables as possible at every meal, so why include just one vegetable when without much more effort you could eat a triple whammy? This dish is great for getting prebiotic leeks into your diet.

2 tbsp extra virgin olive oil
1cm fresh ginger, peeled and grated or chopped
1 garlic clove, peeled and chopped
1 leek, washed and sliced
170g sugar snap peas, thick tips cut off
100g spinach, washed
A splash of tamari sauce

Heat the oil with the ginger and garlic in a pan. Add the leek and stir until softened. Add the sugar snaps and spinach and stir until the spinach is wilted. Add a splash of tamari sauce and serve.

BUTTERNUT SQUASH + SWEET POTATO   ①② SOUP SPRINKLED WITH CHILLI WALNUTS

Serves 4

This recipe is great for boosting your vitamin A levels. It is the orange pigments in these vegetables that contain vitamin A, which is important for building a strong gut lining, as is the chicken stock, which contains collagen. If you haven't got much fresh stock in your fridge, dilute what you have with boiled water; if you don't have any chicken stock at all, you can just use boiled water. The more stock the better, though, not just for the collagen but also because it will make you feel more full than using just water.

For the soup:

3 tbsp extra virgin olive oil

1 red onion, peeled and chopped

1 garlic clove, peeled and chopped

700g chopped butternut squash and sweet potato (you can buy these in bags, ready-chopped, in supermarkets if you need to save time)

500ml fresh chicken stock or water, or a combination of both

Sea salt

Freshly ground black pepper

For the nut topping:

A pinch of sea salt and freshly ground black pepper

Shelled walnut halves (10 per person)

A sprinkle of dried chilli flakes

Sea salt

Heat the olive oil in a pan and sweat the chopped onion and garlic until soft and slightly transparent.

Add the butternut squash and sweet potato and sweat until soft.

Add the stock/water and simmer on a low heat for 20 minutes, partially covered with a lid, until the squash and sweet potato are soft and break up easily when prodded with a fork.

Meanwhile, dry-fry the walnuts, sprinkled with a pinch each of dried chilli flakes and sea salt, until the nuts are warm and fragrant.

Blitz the soup in a blender, then add salt and freshly ground pepper to taste. Sprinkle the nuts over the soup before serving.

ROAST PEPPER + TOMATO SOUP ① ②

Serves 4

You could serve this as a starter in the evening to get your vegetable count up, or as a main meal for lunch, with seeds scattered on top for some protein. If you are in the second fortnight of the plan, crumble over a matchbox-sized piece of Roquefort.

5 large tomatoes
2 red bell peppers or sweet red peppers (the long pointy ones)
2 tbsp extra virgin olive oil
1 small onion, chopped
1 garlic clove, peeled and chopped
400ml fresh chicken stock or water, heated
Sea salt and freshly ground black pepper

Heat the oven to 220°C.

Put the tomatoes and peppers on a baking tray and drizzle over 1 tbsp extra virgin olive oil. Roast in the oven for 20–30 minutes, until the skins are blistering, then remove.

Place the peppers in a cold saucepan with a lid on and leave to cool for about 15 minutes – this helps the skin to loosen and makes them easier to peel. Peel the peppers and remove the seeds and stalks.

When the tomatoes have cooled down a bit, pinch off the skins.

Heat the remaining olive oil in a pan over a medium heat. Add the onions and garlic and sweat them for about 5 minutes. Stir in the peppers and tomatoes. Add the stock (or water if you don't have any real stock) and simmer for 5–10 minutes over a low heat.

Blitz the mixture in a powerful blender, season to taste and serve.

GAZPACHO   ①②

Serves 4

Cold Spanish tomato soup tastes much better than it sounds. It's a kind of Virgin Mary that you can serve as a starter in a cup. Basically it's a liquidised salad – easy to make and it can be stored in the fridge for a couple of days for a quick down-in-one vegetable boost on the run.

400g tinned tomatoes
½ red onion, peeled and chopped
½ medium cucumber
1 garlic clove, peeled and chopped
1 red bell pepper, deseeded and chopped
2 tbsp extra virgin olive oil
1 tbsp red wine vinegar
Sea salt and freshly ground black pepper, to taste
A dash of Tabasco (optional)

Blend all the ingredients in a blender and store in a jug in the fridge until ready to serve. If too thick, you can add a little water, or blend in some ice cubes, for a more soupy consistency.

GERMAN POTATO SALAD   ①②

Serves 4

If you think potato salad is all gloopy mayonnaise dressings, think again. This version from the south of Germany uses vinaigrette instead, and is naturally perfect gut food – it contains not only prebiotic fibres but also fresh chicken stock for the gut lining. It's important you wait until the potatoes have cooled before eating them, because, when cold, potatoes form a type of fibre called resistant starch, which acts as a prebiotic to feed the beneficial bacteria in your gut. Raw onion gives the salad a nice flavour kick but it also acts as another prebiotic. The chicken stock adds collagen and makes the salad fresh and juicy.

Go easy when serving this salad. Spoon it over about a third of your plate, so that you leave room for lots of colour from other vegetables.

750g new potatoes, washed and boiled with skins on until tender
½ white onion, peeled and finely chopped
1 tsp French mustard
4 tbsp extra virgin olive oil
1 tbsp white wine vinegar
½ cup chicken stock (bring this to room temperature if it is jellified from the fridge, so it is in liquid form)
½ tsp sea salt

Slice the potatoes into thin circles and place in a salad bowl.

In another bowl, mix together the onions, mustard, oil, vinegar, stock and salt with a fork, then add this to the potatoes and let it soak in.

This dish goes really well with the Pork Schnitzels (see page 176) and a big half-plateful of steamed fresh asparagus (which also contain its own type of prebiotic fibres).

QUICK TIPS FOR CROWDING OUT GRAINS WITH VEGETABLES

A diet featuring a lot of grains can become an irritant to the gut lining in some people. Many of us eat quite a large volume of grains over the course of a week, but actually little variety of them (i.e. we limit ourselves to just two or three main ones such as wheat, oats, rice). During this month we are taking a holiday from grains, to allow the gut a chance to repair. This provides a big opportunity to use the space left free on the plate, which we would normally fill with grains, with much more nutrient-dense, gut-friendly foods: vegetables that are teeming with plant chemicals, fibre, vitamins and minerals.

1. CAULIFLOWER INSTEAD OF RICE

Cut the hard stalks off a cauliflower and wash and chop the florets into tiny pieces – really shred it, or blitz in a food processor.

Saute the shredded cauliflower in a pan with a drizzle of olive oil until soft, then serve with a pinch of salt. You can add chopped fresh herbs if you like, to make it more tasty, and push up your plant count.

2. COURGETTE INSTEAD OF SPAGHETTI

See Courgette Bolognaise on page 177. You can either spiralize courgettes into the shape of spaghetti, or if you don't have a spiralizer, simply slice them into half moons, sauté them in olive oil and top them with bolognaise sauce.

3. MIXED ROAST VEGETABLES INSTEAD OF COUSCOUS

You can buy mixed ready-chopped vegetables in supermarkets, or you could chop up an array of your favourites and bake them in several trays, drizzled with olive oil, in a medium oven until soft. They are delicious eaten immediately, or at room temperature the next day or in packed lunches.

Roast your favourite chopped veg to get a good combination of colours and flavours; my ideal combination is mushrooms, carrots, cauliflower, parsnips, sweet potato, onion and garlic. Squeeze a lemon over the top before serving with a sprinkle of sea salt for extra taste.

4. USE SWEET POTATOES INSTEAD OF GRAINS

Sweet potatoes contain vitamin A in their orange pigment, which supports your gut lining, so they provide a good nutrient boost instead of grains.

5. USE COLD POTATOES IN MODERATION

Remember, cold potatoes contain resistant starch, which isn't digested in the upper digestive system so it keeps you feeling fuller for longer than hot potatoes. They are useful on one-third of your plate, where you might usually put your grains, but make sure you get lots of colour on the rest of your plate, so there is still a variety of vegetables. We don't want white potatoes becoming the predominant colour, as your gut needs more variety than this.

NIÇOISE SALAD ① ②

Serves 2

For the salad:

1 bag of washed green leaves of your choice

6 cherry tomatoes, halved

3 boiled eggs, quartered

1 tin of tuna in olive oil

1 small bag of flat-leaf parsley, washed and finely chopped

½ red onion, peeled and thinly sliced

100g thin green beans, trimmed, steamed and cooled

2 small cold potatoes

For the dressing:

3 tbsp extra virgin olive oil

1 tbsp freshly squeezed lemon juice or apple cider vinegar

1 garlic clove, roughly chopped

A pinch of sea salt

Toss all the salad ingredients together in a large bowl.

Combine all the dressing ingredients in a cup and stir together well. Pour the dressing over the salad ingredients and serve immediately.

BEETROOT 'HUMMUS' ① ②

This tastes delicious smeared on circles of cucumber. If you're on the second half of the plan, it's great spread on a slice of nut 'bread' with a crumble of Roquefort on top.

4 large beetroots, washed

1 garlic clove, peeled and chopped

Juice of 1 lemon

1 tbsp tahini

Sea salt and freshly ground black pepper, to taste

Heat the oven to 180°C.

Roast the beetroots in the oven for about 1 hour, or until tender. Remove from the oven and leave until cool enough to handle, then peel off the skins.

Put the beetroots with all the other ingredients in a blender and blitz until fully combined and a smooth texture. If you prefer a chunkier texture, you can grate the beetroots and mix them with the other ingredients.

CHICORY STUFFED WITH TUNA   ① ②

Serves 2

This can make a quick self-assembly lunch at home, a great starter or an on-the-go packed lunch (just pack the chicory leaves and the filling in separate plastic pots and assemble them when you are ready to eat).

8 chicory leaves, washed

1 tin of tuna or sardines in olive oil

1 tbsp capers

1 large gherkin, chopped

Juice of ½ lime

2 globe artichokes from a tin or jar

Arrange the chicory leaves on a plate.

Mash all the other ingredients together with a fork, including the olive oil from the tin. Divide the mixture between the chicory leaves and serve.

STIR-FRIED SICHUAN GREEN BEANS ② WITH TEMPEH

Serves 1

Sichuan peppers have many different spellings and names (you might see them called Szechuan peppers, or Sichuan flower peppercorns). They taste lemony/peppery and give your whole mouth a really nice buzz (a bit like pins and needles – but nicer!). They are brilliant for cheering up vegetables or tempeh (the fermented soya you can buy in the fridge section or in jars from health food stores). Sichuan peppers are widely available online and in some supermarkets, such as Sainsbury's. I was first introduced to these peppers by my Chinese sister-in-law Shuang, who comes from Cheng Du in western China, where they are a staple of the local, widely-acclaimed cooking.

200g green beans, topped and tailed
3 tbsp extra virgin olive oil
1 tsp dried chilli flakes
1 tsp Sichuan flower peppercorns, crushed or finely chopped
1 tsp ground ginger
1 garlic clove, peeled and finely chopped
½ small white onion, thinly sliced
4 pieces of tempeh, sliced into small pieces
1 tbsp tamari sauce

Wash the green beans, then lay them on a piece of kitchen roll and make sure they are completely dry.

Heat the oil in a wok or frying pan and cook the beans over a medium heat for about 10 minutes until they are a little crinkled and slightly charred. Remove them from the pan and set aside on a plate.

Add the chilli flakes, flower peppercorns, ginger, garlic and onion to the pan and fry until the onions are melted and moist. Then add the tempeh and stir to coat with the mixture. Toss in the tamari and green beans and serve.

STIR-FRIED PAK CHOI WITH ① ②
SICHUAN PEPPERS

Serves 4

You could serve this as a side dish to boost your vegetable count for the day, or add a handful of cooked prawns or slices of baby squid per person near the end to make it into a main meal.

1 tsp Sichuan peppers flower peppercorns, crushed or finely
   chopped
2cm fresh ginger, peeled and grated
2 garlic cloves, peeled and chopped
1 tbsp coconut oil
6 pak choi, washed, trimmed and leaves separated
4 spring onions, chopped
1 tbsp tamari sauce
1 tbsp fish sauce

Sauté the Sichuan peppers, ginger, and garlic in the coconut oil and cook on a gentle heat until the garlic is moist. Add the pak choi and spring onions and stir until slightly wilted. Add the tamari and fish sauces and serve.

PADRON PEPPERS　　①②

Padron peppers are readily available in supermarkets nowadays and they make a wonderful side dish or starter. Eating this dish is a little like playing Russian roulette with your food – you never know when a hot one will strike!

3 tbsp extra virgin olive oil
130g Padron peppers
¼ tsp sea salt

Heat the oil in a pan over a medium heat, add the Padron peppers whole and stir fry for 5–10 minutes until they are beginning to blister. Serve with sea salt.

CARROT + KEFIR SALAD　　②

Serves 4

I've adapted this recipe from a dish I ate at the Huzur Vadisi yoga retreat in Turkey, where I stayed a few years back in a yurt and ate like royalty for a week. The cooked carrots make this salad delicious and nutritious – cooked carrots deliver higher levels of vitamin A than raw ones, which is good news for your gut lining.

5 large carrots, grated
3 tbsp extra virgin olive oil
½ tsp sea salt
160ml kefir
1 tbsp tahini
A handful of chopped walnuts
2 garlic cloves, peeled and finely chopped

Sauté the grated carrots in the olive oil in a pan over a medium heat until they turn from a bright orange to a more yellowy orange colour. Stir in the salt.

Wait for the mixture to cool then stir in the kefir, tahini, walnuts and garlic and serve at room temperature.

ROASTED BELL PEPPERS   ① ②

Serves 2

Bell peppers are a wonderful source of vitamin C, which is needed to make energy in the body and supports good skin. Plus, if you use a variety of different colours here, you widen the diversity in your diet to help expand your gut flora. However, some individuals find peppers difficult to digest when they are raw or have the skin on. This recipe gets over these issues and the roasting brings out their sweet flavour.

3 bell peppers – red, yellow and green
Drizzle of extra virgin olive oil
Juice of ½ lemon
A pinch of sea salt

Heat the oven to 230°C.

Put the peppers on a baking sheet and bake for 20–30 minutes until the skins are blistering and slightly charred. Remove from the oven and put them in a pan with a lid on for 15–30 minutes (this makes the skins easier to pull off).

Peel the peppers, cut out the core and seeds and slice the flesh into medium-size strips.

Place the peppers in a bowl and drizzle with a little extra virgin olive oil, the lemon juice and a pinch of sea salt.

ROASTED TOMATOES WITH BASIL   ①②

When I get home and I need to get my plant count up with minimal work, this is the dish I whip up!

6 tomatoes on the vine
A drizzle of olive oil
A sprinkle of sea salt
A grind of black pepper
Bunch of fresh basil (optional)

Heat the oven to 230°C.

Put the tomatoes in a baking dish, drizzle with olive oil, salt and pepper and cook in the oven for about 30 minutes, or until the skins are blistering and the tomatoes look juicy. About 10 minutes before the end, chuck the basil leaves on top and leave them in the oven until they go a little crispy. Whip everything out of the oven and serve.

KEFIR SALAD DRESSING   ②

We're using fermented milk kefir as well as Roquefort cheese here, for a delicious bacteria-laden salad dressing.

80ml kefir
Juice of 1 lemon
1 tbsp extra virgin olive oil
A matchbox-sized crumble of Roquefort
A grind of black pepper

Combine all the ingredients in a bowl and mix gently (the cheese can remain a bit crumbled for texture). Pour over any combination of salad.

PERUVIAN CEVICHE ①②

Serves 4

When I was 19 I went to Lima, Peru, for six months to learn Spanish. At first I was repulsed by the idea of eating raw fish, then I found I craved it when I got back home. In Peru there were cevicherías – informal eateries serving nothing but ceviche – all over the place, with ceviche piled high with red onions, limes and chillies, which 'cook' the raw fish. If you like sushi or sashimi and wasabi, you will probably love ceviche.

When I got back from Peru, in 1989, I couldn't find an English cookbook that included this dish or knew of restaurants serving it. Now ceviche is mega popular in big cities and there are English language cookbooks with dozens of versions. This is mine; it's *Gut Makeover* friendly and makes a brilliant dinner-party dish. A nice accompaniment to this dish is some corn on the cobs drizzled in a little butter (if on phase 2) and salt.

4 pieces of the freshest white fish you can find (about 200g each),
    boned and skinned (I usually use cod)
Juice of 6 limes
Juice of 2 lemons
2 Scotch bonnet peppers, deseeded (or regular fresh chillies of
    your choice)
1 medium red onion, finely sliced into half moons
A small bunch of coriander, roughly chopped

1 tbsp sea salt (yes, 1 tablespoon – it gives it a frozen margarita
  kind of twist)

To serve:

6 sweet potatoes, roasted in their skins for about 1 hour or until
  soft and juicy, then peeled and chopped in half

Essential kit: a really sharp knife.

Lay the pieces of fish on plastic trays/Tupperware lids, or plates and place in the freezer for 1 hour. Whip them out when they are firm, but not frozen through – this makes it easier to cut precise thin slivers. (It's worth planning ahead to include this step – if you don't do this and/or your knife isn't sharp, you can end up with fluffy, rough bits of fish rather than sashimi-style slivers.)

Slice the fish into thin wafers, put them in a bowl and stir in all the remaining ingredients. Within 15 minutes the fish should take on a white 'cooked' appearance.

Serve as soon as possible (marinating the fish for too long can make it mushy). To serve, place the bowl of ceviche in the middle of a platter surrounded with the room-temperature sweet potatoes and, if using, room-temperature cobs of corn. The sweet potatoes are the perfect antidote to the sharp, spicy, citrus flavours of the fish.

BAKED SALMON WITH MUSTARD +   ① ②
ALMOND CRUST

Serves 2

This is ultra quick and easy to make, and it is also quite an economical dish if you use frozen fish. This is delicious with a big pile of mixed greens.

2 organic or wild salmon fillets (defrosted if frozen)
2 tbsp French mustard
2 tbsp flaked almonds
A pinch of sea salt
A drizzle of olive oil

Heat the oven to 200°C.

Put the salmon on a baking tray. Smear mustard on top of each fillet, scatter over the flaked almonds and salt and drizzle over a little olive oil. (This is particularly important if you are using wild Alaskan salmon, as this can be more dry than other types.) The almonds should stick on to form a nice crust when cooked. Bake in the oven for 20 minutes, or until cooked through.

QUICK STEAK DINNER   ① ②

Serves 1

You can vary the steak you use here – organic beef or buffalo, or, if you can get hold of it, use a wild meat such as venison (now sold in supermarkets in fillets, either fresh or frozen). To get some colour on your plate, serve this with a pile of mixed roasted vegetables, or a large heap of chicory salad.

If you have a large steak or prefer to cook more than one at the same time, you can keep any leftovers in the fridge for the Thai salad (see page 169) the next day.

1 tbsp extra virgin olive oil, ghee or butter (if phase 2)
½ onion, peeled and thinly sliced
1 fillet of organic steak – e.g. beef, buffalo or wild venison
A pinch of sea salt
A grind of black pepper

Melt the oil or fat in a frying pan. Add the onion and fry gently until soft and cooked through. Add the steak and sauté gently on both sides until cooked to your liking – you can serve it either raw in the middle or cooked through, depending on your preference. Season with salt and pepper and serve drizzled with the onion and juices from the pan.

THAI BEEF SALAD ①②

Serves 2

The beauty of a salad like this is that it gets a good variety of vegetables into you in one go, including anti-inflammatory herbs, and also whacks in raw garlic and onion, too, which are prebiotic and powerful gut flora boosters. The lemons help with production of stomach acid to aid digestion and absorption of nutrients. Make sure you eat this dish slowly and chew the meat really well.

1 tbsp olive oil

240g organic beef steak (such as sirloin), sprinkled with a pinch of salt

24 cherry tomatoes, halved

½ cucumber, chopped

½ red onion, peeled and sliced

1 green chilli pepper, chopped, or a red one if you like it hotter

2 garlic cloves, peeled and chopped

28g fresh coriander (a largish handful), leaves and stalks washed and finely chopped

1 tbsp fish sauce

1 tsp tamari sauce

Juice of 2 limes

A few fresh mint leaves, torn (optional)

Heat the olive oil in a frying pan over a medium heat and sauté the steak on both sides. Try not to overcook it – leave it slightly rare in the middle if you like your meat juicy.

When it is cooked to your liking, put the steak on a chopping board and, with a sharp knife, cut off the fat and slice the steak into strips.

While the steak is cooling, put the tomatoes, cucumbers, onion, chilli, garlic and herbs into a salad bowl. Add the steak and pour over the fish sauce, tamari and lime juice.

Tip the pan juices over the salad, mmm.

LEMON + ROSEMARY ROASTED CHICKEN ①②

Serves 4

If you have dismissed the idea of buying a whole organic chicken in the past because you think it is too expensive, think again. You get a lot more for your money if you buy a whole chicken rather than breast fillets. You can get maximum value out of one bird by cooking this and the next four recipes.

1 organic chicken
A bunch of fresh rosemary
½ lemon
3 tbsp olive oil
A pinch of sea salt
A grind of black pepper

Heat the oven to 160°C.

Remove any elastic bands or string from the chicken. (You want to be able to get the olive oil and herbs into all the crevices to maximise flavour.) Strip the rosemary leaves off the stalks with your hands, then chop them quite finely.

Put the chicken in a roasting tin, then lightly squeeze the lemon juice over and put the squeezed lemon inside the chicken's cavity. This is key to a juicy, delicious chicken, rather than one that is rubbery and dried out.

Add the rosemary to the olive oil in a small bowl with the salt and pepper. Now pour this over the chicken and massage it into the whole body, especially the legs and wings. This stops the chicken becoming dry when cooking.

Put the chicken in the oven to roast. After 90 minutes, test the chicken to see if it is done – pierce the thigh with the tip of a sharp knife and if the juices run clear, the chicken is cooked. When the chicken is ready, remove it from the oven and leave it to rest for 15 minutes, covered with a piece of tinfoil.

When serving the chicken, make sure each portion comes drizzled with a generous scoop of the delicious lemon/rosemary-flavoured gelatinous juices, which should have formed at the bottom of the pan.

REAL CHICKEN STOCK   ① ②

Makes at least 1 litre

1 chicken carcass and bones, meat picked off

1 litre filtered water

1 celery stick, washed

1 carrot, washed, topped and tailed

1 onion, peeled

2 bay leaves

Put the chicken carcass and bones in a large saucepan and add enough of the water to completely cover the chicken, but do not fill the pan too much or the stock may turn out too watery. Add the celery, carrot, onion and bay leaves.

Bring to the boil, then simmer with the lid on for 3–4 hours, or cook it for half an hour in a pressure cooker. Leave the stock to cool, then pour it through a sieve and discard the bones and vegetables. Pour the clear stock into several containers (I usually divide into four/five plastic containers' worth from the bones of one chicken).

You can keep the stock in the fridge for 4–5 days or freeze it and defrost when needed. If you like, you can pour the stock into an ice-cube tray to give you smaller portions that you can pop out, a few at a time, when needed to go into soups, stir-fries and potato salads.

WARM GREEN CHICKEN SALAD   ① ②

Serves 1

Pouring a warm red onion and red wine vinegar dressing over this salad gives it a delightfully sweet and sour flavour.

2 huge handfuls of baby spinach leaves, washed

A huge handful of rocket leaves, washed

½ tin of anchovies in olive oil, drained and chopped

The leftover chicken picked off the leg of a roast chicken

3 tbsp olive oil

1 red onion, peeled and chopped

2 large garlic cloves, peeled and chopped

2 tbsp red wine vinegar

Combine the salad leaves, anchovies and chicken in a salad bowl.

Heat the olive oil in a pan over a medium heat, add the onion and garlic and sauté until they are soft and slightly transparent. Take off the heat, wait a minute, then add the red wine vinegar. Pour this mixture over the salad and serve at once.

MULTI-COLOURED MISO CHICKEN STIR-FRY ②

Serves 2

Fermented miso – the paste, not the freeze-dried stuff – is a good alternative probiotic food if you can't tolerate kefir.

3 tbsp extra virgin olive oil
1 garlic clove, peeled and chopped
2cm fresh ginger, peeled and chopped
450g bag of vegetable stir-fry mix (available in supermarkets ready-chopped, e.g. beansprouts, broccoli, onions, cabbage, carrots)
1 courgette, sliced (to add bulk, remember no rice!)
A handful of chopped chicken from your leftover roast chicken
1 cup fresh chicken stock (see page 171)
1 tbsp fish sauce
A sprinkle of tamari sauce
1 tbsp fermented miso

Heat the oil into a frying pan and stir fry the garlic and ginger on a medium heat for about two minutes. Add all the vegetables and stir for about five minutes. Add the chicken and chicken stock and stir in.

Cook, stirring occasionally, until the broccoli is al dente (not rock hard, but not limp).

Sprinkle on the fish sauce and tamari to taste, then stir in the miso and serve.

ASIAN-STYLE GUT-HEALING SOUP ②

Serves 1

This is perfect for phase 1 of the plan because chicken stock provides collagen which can help heal the gut lining, and the salmon contains omega-3 essential fatty acids to help reduce gut inflammation (if this is an issue). The pak choi (prebiotic) and fermented miso (probiotic) work in concert to boost gut flora. The first time you try the miso, you may like to start with a quarter teaspoon, or a half, and build up the amount as your gut gets used to it.

A knob of coconut oil
1 garlic clove, peeled and chopped
1cm fresh ginger, peeled and chopped
2 spring onions, sliced
120g organic or wild salmon, cubed
2 pak choi, washed and sliced
1 tsp fresh fermented miso (found in the fridge of good health
    food stores and Asian supermarkets)
250ml fresh chicken stock (see page 171)
Juice of 1 lime
1 tsp tamari sauce
1 tsp fish sauce

Heat the coconut oil in a frying pan or wok on medium heat and sauté the garlic, ginger and spring onions. Add the salmon and cook through. Add the pak choi and stir around until just beginning to wilt. Add the rest of the ingredients and simmer for a few minutes, then serve.

LEBANESE LEMON CHICKEN LIVERS + ① ② POMEGRANATE

Serves 2

I'm always looking for quick, easy and palatable ways to cook organ meats and I came across this combination in a Lebanese restaurant while on holiday in Egypt. Liver contains a form of vitamin A needed to build a strong gut lining, and this form is more absorbable than the type found in the orange pigment of vegetables such as butternut squash and pumpkins. This form is also found in egg yolks and real butter. Some supermarkets now sell organic livers and also pomegranate molasses in bottles.

4 tbsp olive oil
1 red onion, peeled and thinly sliced in half moons
1 garlic clove, peeled and sliced
400g organic chicken livers
1 knob of butter (if on second part of the programme)
2 tbsp pomegranate molasses
Juice of 1 lemon
A sprinkle of sea salt and freshly ground black pepper, to taste
50g fresh watercress

Heat the oil in a pan on a medium heat and gently sauté the onions and garlic until soft. Add the livers and sauté gently – if you want them tender and slightly pink in the middle, whip them off the heat soon after they change colour; if you like them cooked through, leave them slightly longer, but just a couple more minutes otherwise they can become tough. If you're on the second part of the programme, stir in the butter when the livers are cooked.

Stir in the pomegranate molasses then add the lemon juice, salt and pepper.

Pile the watercress leaves onto a plate, top with the livers, then pour the juices over and enjoy.

PORK SCHNITZELS ①②

Serves 4

This is great with two other gut-boosting accompaniments – the German Potato Salad on page 155, and a pile of steamed asparagus. If you are buying your meat from a butcher, ask him or her to stamp each fillet with a meat tenderiser hammer so they are nice and thin and the meat is more tender and easy to digest. If you are buying the meat in a supermarket ready packaged, you could use the steaks as they come (about 1cm thick), or buy a meat tenderiser (about £5) and hammer them yourself to make them less chewy.

English mustard bought as a paste normally contains gluten but the powder doesn't, so it's OK to use in this recipe. Arrowroot is usually found in the baking section of supermarkets.

200g ground almonds (you can buy ready ground)
1 tsp English mustard powder
2 tbsp arrowroot
1 tsp paprika

½ tsp cayenne pepper

1 tsp sea salt

120ml extra virgin olive oil

4 organic pork loin steaks (total weight 500g)

Heat the oven to 220°C.

Combine the ground almonds, mustard powder, arrowroot, paprika, cayenne pepper and sea salt in a shallow bowl.

Pour the olive oil into a separate shallow bowl.

Dip each piece of pork into the oil then dip it into the almond mixture to coat it on both sides. Place on a baking tray and cook the schnitzels in the oven for 20 minutes until golden brown.

COURGETTE BOLOGNAISE   ① ②

Serves 8

I've been cooking this for years, first in a big pot, which would hiss and steam on the hob for hours, but more recently in a pressure cooker in just half an hour. Don't limit yourself to beef for tradition's sake; it's important to use a variety of proteins in the diet to expose ourselves to a range of different nutrients, so go beyond beef in your bolognaise. Minced meat should be easy to digest and absorb because not only has it been minced, as the name suggests, but it has been well cooked, too.

If you make it in bulk, like this, you can freeze leftovers in small portions for another day.

4 tbsp extra virgin olive oil

1 large onion (or 2 small ones), peeled and finely chopped

4 garlic cloves, peeled and chopped

2 celery sticks, finely chopped

1kg organic beef, buffalo or lamb mince

800g whole plum tomatoes, tinned (I prefer whole to chopped as I find they retain more flavour)

140g tomato purée

4 tbsp fresh chicken stock

A bunch of fresh rosemary, washed and leaves chopped finely

1 tsp sea salt

Heat the oil in a pan (or pressure cooker pot if you prefer) on a medium heat and sauté the onion, garlic and celery. Add the mince and cook until browned, stirring occasionally.

Add the tomatoes and tomato purée, chicken stock, rosemary and salt and stir, gently breaking up the plum tomatoes with a wooden spoon.

Cook on a low heat with the lid slightly ajar for 3–4 hours, or cook according to the manufacturer's instructions for 30 minutes in a pressure cooker.

For the courgette 'spaghetti':

1 medium courgette per person

2 tbsp extra virgin olive oil

A pinch of sea salt

Top and tail the courgettes and turn them through a spiralizer. If you don't have a spiralizer, slice the courgettes into half moons. Put a tablespoon of olive oil in a pan, add the courgettes and cook for a few minutes until softened – half moon shapes may need a little longer. Season with a pinch of sea salt.

Serve the spaghetti on individual plates, topped with a portion of bolognaise sauce.

MEDITERRANEAN ROAST VEGETABLES ① ②

Serves 2

This is a good way of filling a large portion of your plate with a variety of different vegetables. The combination here is just a suggestion – you probably have your own favourites. If you're short of time, you can cheat by buying bags of ready-chopped vegetables from supermarkets and roasting them drizzled with a little olive oil and sea salt.

1 large red onion, peeled and cut into eighths
1 large courgette, trimmed, cut into three widthways, then eighths
  lengthways
1 yellow pepper, seeded and cut into eighths
20 cherry tomatoes
4 tbsp olive oil
A sprinkle of sea salt and freshly ground black pepper, to taste

Heat the oven to 160°C.
  Tip all the ingredients into a roasting tin and mix together well. Slow-roast in the oven for 50 minutes until softened and juicy.

LAZY LAMB CURRY ① ②

Serves 8

A curry like this, where the meat has been really well cooked, is important for easy digestion and the absorption of important nutrients from the meat. This dish also includes a good whack of chicken stock to provide collagen for your gut lining, and ginger and turmeric, which are both powerful anti-inflammatories

– good for an inflamed digestive system or for post-exercise aches and pains. It is a really low-work dish.

2 tbsp extra virgin olive oil

1kg organic lamb fillet, cut into cubes

2 white onions, peeled and chopped

3 large garlic cloves, peeled and chopped

1–2 chillies (depending on how spicy you like your curry), finely chopped

1 tbsp fresh ginger, peeled and chopped

1 tbsp turmeric, either freshly grated or ground, plus extra to serve

1 tbsp garam masala

1 tbsp ground cumin

800g tinned chopped tomatoes

300ml fresh chicken stock

400ml coconut milk

240g baby spinach leaves, washed

1 tsp sea salt

Sweat and stir the first nine ingredients in a pan for about 5 minutes on a medium heat.

Add the tomatoes and the chicken stock, then turn the heat down and put a lid on the pan. Leave to simmer for 3–4 hours. If you prefer, you could cook this in a pressure cooker in just 30 minutes.

When the meat is tender and soft, stir in the coconut milk, baby spinach and sea salt. The spinach should just wilt into the mixture – take the pan off the heat after a couple of minutes before the spinach becomes mushy.

Serve with cauliflower rice (see box on page 157) sprinkled with turmeric.

LAMB SHANK TAGINE + FIVE VEGETABLES ① ②

Serves 8

If you get your hands on some lamb shanks, it's an opportunity to cook up a feast that hopefully will last several meals and provide more for the freezer. When I went to Morocco, I loved the preserved lemon and pomegranate molasses that give dishes a sweet and sour edge, so I've used both in this recipe. Increasingly, supermarkets are selling Moroccan ingredients such as these, and they are also widely available online.

I've adopted the tradition here of serving the tagine with large pieces of steamed vegetables as a chance to load up on vegetables. Cooking this should also leave you with a jug of lamb stock, which can be used as a base for cooking soups in future.

For the meat and stock:

4 lamb shanks
4 garlic cloves
A generous grind of black pepper
About 750ml water

For the sauce:

2 tbsp extra virgin olive oil
1 small red onion, peeled and sliced into thin moons
1 garlic clove, peeled and chopped
1cm fresh ginger, peeled and grated
1 tsp ras-el-hanout
½ tsp sweet paprika
½ tsp turmeric
½ tsp cumin

½ tsp cinnamon

400g tin plum tomatoes

1 tsp honey

2 tbsp pomegranate molasses

3 preserved lemons, pips removed and chopped

A handful of blanched whole almonds

A handful of green olives, pitted

Sea salt (optional) and freshly ground black pepper

For the vegetables:

Any or all of:

1 pointy cabbage, washed and sliced into four

1 swede, peeled and cubed

1 sweet potato, peeled and cubed

1 butternut squash, peeled and cubed

1 courgette, cut into quarters

Put the shanks, meaty side down, in an ovenproof casserole dish with the garlic and black pepper. Pour in enough of the water to cover the main meaty parts, and gently simmer in the oven (160°C) with the lid on, until the meat is falling off the bone (about 3 hours). Alternatively, cook on a low heat on the hob for about 3 hours, or in a pressure cooker for 35 minutes.

Remove the shanks and drain the water, which should now look like a nice golden stock, into another container and leave to cool. Pick the meat off the bones, then remove and discard any large pieces of fat.

To make the sauce, heat the oil in a pan on a medium heat and sauté the onion and garlic until soft. Stir in the ginger and spices. Add the tomatoes, honey, molasses and preserved lemons and heat gently, stirring occasionally so the sauce does not stick on the bottom of the pan. Now add the tender meat, stripped from the bones, to the sauce.

Before serving, add the almonds and olives, and season with a little salt, if needed, and pepper. The lemons and olives can be quite salty already, so judge if you need extra.

Meanwhile, steam the vegetables of your choice. Serve the tagine mixture on top of, or alongside, the vegetables.

Store the lamb stock in the fridge to use in soups and stir fries. It makes a good alternative to chicken stock, and contains many of the same benefits.

MEATBALLS IN PAPRIKA + CAYENNE ① ②
TOMATO SAUCE

Serves 4

Meatballs make a hearty meal and are often good heated or eaten at room temperature again the next day. If you set some meatballs aside after cooking them and don't add sauce, you can keep these as a convenient protein addition to an easy-to-eat packed lunch.

500g minced meat (lamb, beef, pork or a mixture of two of these)
A handful of fresh flat-leaf parsley, chopped
1 egg
4 garlic cloves, peeled and finely chopped
1 tsp smoked sweet paprika

For the sauce:

2 tbsp extra virgin olive oil
4 red onions, peeled and finely chopped
1 garlic clove, peeled and finely chopped

2 tsp cayenne pepper
1 tsp smoked sweet paprika
800g whole plum tomatoes, tinned
Sea salt and freshly ground black pepper

Heat the oven to 200°C.

Mix the meat, parsley, egg, garlic and sweet paprika in a bowl. Put spoonfuls into the palm of your hand and roll them into balls or small patties.

Place them on a baking tray in rows, slightly spaced apart, and bake for about 20 minutes, until cooked through.

Meanwhile, make the sauce. Heat the olive oil in a pan on a medium heat and sauté the onion and garlic for 5 minutes, then add the cayenne pepper, paprika and plum tomatoes, breaking up the tomatoes with a spoon. Season to taste and leave to simmer for 15 minutes.

When the meatballs are done, add them to the sauce and cook for 5 minutes. Serve with a large green salad with avocados and nuts.

SPANISH MEATBALLS IN ALMOND SAUCE ①②

Serves 4

We normally think about meatballs going well with tomato sauces, but almond sauces, which are popular in Spanish cooking, are delicious, and nutritious, too.

500g minced pork
1 small onion, finely chopped
1 garlic clove, peeled and finely chopped

½ tsp sea salt

Freshly ground black pepper, to taste

A powdering of grated nutmeg

1 egg

1 tbsp ground almonds

3 tbsp extra virgin olive oil

For the almond sauce:

3 tbsp olive oil

2 garlic cloves, peeled and finely chopped

4 tbsp ground almonds

1 tsp hot smoked paprika

½ tsp ground black pepper

½ tsp salt

200ml thick, gelatinous chicken stock (add a little water if you
   need to make the sauce a little thinner)

Put all the meatball ingredients, except the olive oil, in a bowl
and mix them together. Put spoonfuls into the palm of your hand
and roll them into small balls.

Heat the olive oil in a pan on a medium heat, add the meatballs and pan-fry until they are lightly browned. Keep turning
them every couple of minutes so they cook through properly. Set
aside and make the almond sauce.

In a clean pan, heat the olive oil on a medium heat. Add the
garlic and fry until golden, then add the ground almonds, hot
smoked paprika, salt and pepper. Stir in the chicken stock then
add the meatballs. Leave on a low heat for about 5 minutes while
the sauce thickens.

SEA BASS WITH SALSA VERDE ① ②

Serves 4

This is an ultra-quick meal for after work and provides good leftovers, too! The salsa verde can be used the next day to accompany other dishes or as a dressing for a salad, thinned down with more extra virgin olive oil.

The fish:

4 sea bass fillets with skin on
1 tbsp extra virgin olive oil
A pinch of sea salt
A grind of black pepper

The sauce:

A handful of basil
A handful of parsley
1 tbsp capers
4 tinned anchovy fillets
4 tbsp extra virgin olive oil
1 tbsp Dijon mustard
1 garlic clove, peeled and chopped

Place all the sauce ingredients in a blender and blitz in short bursts until the main ingredients are broken down, but the mixture is still rough and textured. Set aside.

Lightly season the fish. Heat the oil in a frying pan over a medium heat then place the fish skin-side down in the pan and cook over a medium heat until the skin is crispy. Turn over and cook for a couple of minutes on the other side until cooked through.

Serve the fish with a drizzle of the salsa verde on top and a large portion of green salad or steamed spinach on the side.

BUN-LESS BURGER + SWEET POTATO WEDGES ①②

Serves 4

When it comes to burgers, I'm a great believer in simplicity and quality. That's why the meat speaks for itself here and the condiments sing the chorus. The wedges can be dunked in the raw tomato ketchup on page 192.

For the burger:

500g beef or buffalo mince
½ small white onion, finely chopped
A small handful of fresh flat-leaf parsley, finely chopped
1 egg
Sea salt and freshly ground black pepper, to taste
Extra virgin olive oil, for frying
A small slice of Roquefort cheese per burger (phase 2)
4 slices of gherkin
1 tomato, sliced

For the wedges:

4 medium-sized sweet potatoes, peeled and cut into wedges
4 tbsp extra virgin olive oil
A sprinkle of cayenne pepper
A sprinkle of paprika
½ tsp sea salt

Heat the oven to 200°C.

First get the potatoes in the oven. Lay the wedges on a large oven tray and sprinkle with the oil, cayenne pepper, paprika and salt. Stir the ingredients together with your hands or a spoon so they are all coated in the mixture. Cook in the oven for 40 minutes or until golden. Halfway through the cooking time, take the potatoes out and tussle them around so the other sides are exposed and can crisp up.

While the potatoes are cooking, make the burgers. Using a wooden spoon, mix the meat with the onion, parsley, egg and salt and pepper to taste, then split the mixture into four and form into round burger shapes with your hands.

Put a little olive oil in a frying pan, cook the burgers on a medium heat for about 5 minutes, until they are lightly browned, then turn them over and keep cooking until they are cooked through. Near the end, put a slice of Roquefort on top and let it melt into the top of the burger (phase 2 only).

Serve a burger on each plate with a slice of tomato and gherkin on top and the sweet potato wedges on the side. Serve with the raw ketchup on page 192.

GUT MAKEOVER 'BREAD' ① ②

I thought long and hard before including this recipe, as nuts and seeds eaten in bulk can mean a large amount of fat in one sitting. Although *The Gut Makeover* includes beneficial fats as needed in cooking to make it taste good, and to make us feel full, they do need to be kept in check, so a meal isn't dominated by them.

We're aiming for the vegetables and colour to take centre stage in every meal, so enjoy a slice of this toasted, with a smear of miso paste on top, or some roasted artichokes from a jar, or some beetroot hummus, or with roasted peppers and a squeeze of lemon and maybe a little cayenne pepper, and a large side salad, to keep your plant count up. This recipe is an adaptation from one by Danish celebrity chef Thomas Rode.

3 cups walnuts, roughly chopped
2 cups almonds, roughly chopped
2 cups mixed seeds, e.g. pumpkin seeds, sunflower seeds,
    flaxseeds
5 eggs, beaten
80ml extra virgin olive oil, plus extra for oiling the loaf tin
1 tsp sea salt

Heat the oven to 160°C.

Mix the nuts and seeds together in a bowl. In another bowl, mix together the eggs, oil and sea salt. Stir the wet and dry ingredients together.

Decant the mixture into a loaf tin greased with olive oil and bake in the oven for 1 hour. Remove from the oven and leave to cool in the tin.

Leave to cool before cutting into slices.

When cooled, store wrapped, in a fridge, to keep it fresh longer.

How to assemble a *Gut Makeover* packed lunch

Many of the recipes in this book provide great leftovers for lunch the next day – anything from curry with cauliflower rice to Bolognaise with courgette spaghetti. Sometimes slow-cooked foods just taste even better the next day.

If you have a microwave or oven at work you could heat up the leftovers for lunch – if you are using a microwave, empty your lunch onto a ceramic plate first and heat on this to avoid microwaved plastic leaching into your food.

I prefer my packed lunches at room temperature; in most UK weather, you don't need to worry about your food going off between coming out of your fridge in the morning and being eaten five hours later at lunch.

All of the following lunch ideas can be eaten cold or at room temperature. See the section below on dressings, dips and sauces if you want to jazz up these dishes.

It's a good idea to invest in some portable, non-spill containers to transport your lunch in. Choose a box with a lid for the main ingredients below and a separate, smaller, lidded one for sauces, dips or dressings.

Protein	Load up with plants
Smoked mackerel – bought ready to eat	Ready-cooked beetroots + washed chicory leaves go really well with this. Add French dressing and a small, cold white potato.
Steak	Bag of mixed salad leaves (the more varieties the better, e.g. lamb's lettuce, rocket and watercress). A small, cold white potato. A drizzle of pesto, mixed with extra virgin olive oil, over the lot.
Roast chicken leg	A big pile of roasted vegetables. The raw ketchup goes nicely with these and the meat.
2 boiled eggs and ½ tin of tuna and some anchovies	Chopped tomatoes, cucumbers, red onions, Kalamata olives and a vinaigrette dressing.
Wild Alaskan salmon	Sliced ripe avocado, pieces of celery and radishes and a drizzle of extra virgin olive oil and a teaspoon of balsamic vinegar.
Pork schnitzel	German potato salad + a large pile of steamed green asparagus.

Bring a piece of fruit for dessert or as a starter, as this automatically bumps up your plant count for the day.

Dressings, dips and sauces

Some people say they don't eat many vegetables each day because they find them boring or not particularly tasty. The way to jazz up vegetables and make sure they taste good is to have delicious dressings, dips and sauces to hand. They often provide the bridge to vegetables and hence a better diet. Here are three simple additions that can be easily be put together to liven up most lunch box combinations.

1. **Pesto** – Put into a powerful blender: a large handful of fresh basil leaves, about 80ml of extra virgin olive oil, the juice of a lemon, a handful of pine nuts and a little salt. Make it quite runny so it acts as a nice cold sauce you can drizzle over cold meats, fish and salads or roast vegetables.

2. **Raw ketchup** – Put into a powerful blender: half a jar of sun-dried tomatoes (about 150ml – you can buy them in jars, packed in olive oil) with two tablespoons of extra virgin olive oil, two large fresh tomatoes, half a red onion, a garlic clove, a handful of fresh basil and a little sea salt. Add enough olive oil to make the sauce the consistency of tomato ketchup. This is absolutely delicious and great for the gut flora because the onions and garlic are raw rather than cooked.

3. **Simple French dressing** – Stir together three parts extra virgin olive oil to one part red wine vinegar with a teaspoon of French mustard and a little sea salt and pepper. The mustard not only tastes good but binds the other ingredients together.

WARNING: Healthy behaviours are infectious

I recently worked with a company of 40 staff in London on a workplace wellness programme. The CEO was proud that her staff represented 15 different nationalities, the point being that talent was recruited from all over the world, and the company was a culturally rich place to work. I noticed immediately that around 80 per cent of the staff were bringing in delicious leftovers, from multi-coloured, vegetable-count-high curries to bolognaise, and eating them at tables in a communal kitchen. These staff members were not only saving money by doing this but supporting their health, too.

So the starting point for improving this group's eating habits was several notches above anywhere else I have been, where the status quo is often poor-quality sandwiches eaten at desks. Infectious behaviours are important when it comes to developing healthy behaviours; if you work around others who are eating low-nutrient, beige-coloured food at their desks, you are more likely to do so too. If you hang around with people who cook proper evening meals and bring in leftovers the next day and move away from their desks to eat it, you are also likely to – and others may even join you!

I recommend doing *The Gut Makeover* with a buddy if you can find one. You can support one another, but you may also find your new eating habits and behaviours start to spread to other colleagues, too.

Sample meal plans

A weekend – phase ① or ②

	Saturday	Sunday
Breakfast	Spinach scrambled egg + glass of green gunge Ginger tea	Wild salmon + avocado + glass of green gunge Ginger tea
Lunch	Fillet of smoked cooked mackerel, cooked beetroot, chicory leaves and French dressing A banana	Roast chicken with lemon and olive oil with roasted vegetables + a corn on the cob
Dinner	Bowl of butternut squash/sweet potato soup with roasted walnuts Half a mango	Mario's orange-onion-olive salad + tin of sardines in olive oil A cup of gazpacho
Remember at each meal:	Sit down, slow down, chew properly	Sit down, slow down, chew properly

On Saturday, if this plan is executed properly, you should consume seven American cup sizes of plants – five as vegetables and two as fruit. Just so you can start to see what this looks like:

1 cup spinach (in eggs)
1 cup kale, orange, ginger, etc. (in green gunge)
1 cup beetroot
1 cup chicory
1 banana = 1 cup
1 cup pumpkin/butternut squash
1 cup mango

On Sunday:
1 cup avocado
1 cup of various in green gunge
2 cups in roast vegetables, e.g. squash, mushrooms, cauliflower
1 cup sweetcorn
1 orange in the salad
1 cup in the gazpacho

You'll see we have covered around 14 different types of vegetables and fruit in this list. We are aiming to eat 20–30 different plants a week (the wider the diversity of plants, the wider the diversity of gut flora and the better it is for your health). This weekend plan means we are more than halfway there on variety for the week already.

If you have a large appetite or are of a larger build and need more nutrition, you could even ramp up the plants to another portion or two a day, e.g. you could have 2 cups of squash on Sunday, as they will melt down when baked, and you could add in another cup of pumpkin and have more soup on the Saturday.

A week in phase ①

Monday	Tuesday	Wednesday	Thursday	Friday	Varieties
Banana nut bread + small green gunge	Ripe sliced avocado + wild salmon	Scrambled eggs + wild salmon + green gunge	Nutty non-dairy shake	Banana nut bread + small green gunge	Banana Kale Orange Ginger Mint Red onion
Leftover chicken + roast vegetables	Leftover bolognaise + spiralized courgettes	Gut-healing Asian soup	Lazy lamb curry + cauliflower rice	Niçoise salad	Courgette Yellow pepper Cherry tomatoes Apple Tomatoes
Piece of fruit	Piece of fruit	Piece of fruit	Piece of fruit	Piece of fruit	Garlic Plum Avocado
Bolog-naise + spiralized courgettes	Multi-coloured stir-fry + squash soup	Lazy lamb curry + cauliflower 'rice'	Warm green chicken salad + roast pepper and tomato soup	Baked salmon with mustard + almond crust with triple greens	Kiwi Beansprouts Cabbage Carrots Pear Spring onions Pak choi Lime Cauliflower
Mixed greens side salad		Mixed greens side salad		Small side of roast veg.	Turmeric Spinach Melon Blueberries
Remember at each meal: Sit down, slow down, chew properly					Rocket Strawberries Parsley Olives Nectarine Lemon Leeks Sugar snaps
7 cups	7 cups	7 cups	7 cups	7 cups	35 varieties

A week in phase ②, if you can tolerate dairy

Monday	Tuesday	Wednesday	Thursday	Friday
Kefir berry/ banana shake	Kefir pineapple shake	Kefir berry/ banana shake	Kefir pineapple shake	Kefir berry/ banana shake
Thai organic beef salad	Chicory, pine nut and Roquefort salad	Niçoise salad	Leftover pork schnitzel + German potato salad + steamed asparagus	Roast Mediterranean vegetables omelette
Piece of fruit	Piece of fruit	Piece of fruit	Piece of fruit	Piece of fruit or a cup of gazpacho
Butternut squash/ sweet potato soup + sautéed chilli walnuts	Pork schnitzel + German potato salad + steamed asparagus	Lebanese lemon chicken livers + watercress	Warm green chicken salad	Ceviche with red onions, sweet potatoes + corn on the cob

Remember at each meal: Sit down, slow down, chew properly

A week in phase ② , if you are non-dairy:

Monday	Tuesday	Wednesday	Thursday	Friday
Banana nut bread + small green gunge	Ripe sliced avocado + wild salmon	Scrambled eggs + wild salmon + a piece of fruit	Nutty non-dairy shake	Banana nut bread + small green gunge
Warm chicken salad	Chicory + apple salad + walnuts	Leftover pork schnitzel + German potato salad + steamed asparagus	Leftover roast vegetables + pumpkin seeds	Leftover chicken livers + pile of watercress with dressing
Butternut squash/ sweet potato soup + sautéed chilli walnuts	Pork schnitzel + German potato salad + steamed asparagus	Roast mixed vegetables with handful of roasted pumpkin seeds	Lebanese lemon chicken livers on a pile of rocket leaves	Piece of smoked mackerel + German potato salad + 2 bought cooked beetroots, chopped
Piece of fruit	Piece of fruit	Piece of fruit	Piece of fruit	Piece of fruit

Remember at each meal: Sit down, slow down, chew properly

PART FOUR

Eating for life

Introduction

I hope by now you've lost some weight, your skin is glowing and you're feeling brighter all round. Your *Gut Makeover* is complete! And now you're wondering how you can maintain your happy digestive system and continue to look and feel good for the long term.

That is what this chapter is about.

This plan is nutrient-dense, anti-inflammatory and easy to follow going forward. Keep eating in this style and you shouldn't suffer a sugar, alcohol or gluten craving! You'll also get your calcium from an abundance of green leafy vegetables, some nuts and seeds, and the kefir and Roquefort. Carbohydrates are contained in vegetables and fruits, so you can get energy from plants rather than traditional grains.

If you have a large amount of weight to lose and you're in the full swing of the plan – enjoying the benefits of a healthier gut, not feeling hungry and relishing having plenty of energy while the weight is dropping off, probably half a kilo a week – then you can carry on until you reach your target weight. Look in your diary and plan another month, then review it again if you continue, or decide to carry on eating this way after that.

If you do decide to go on longer, the rest of this chapter may be more relevant when you are ready to move on to the maintenance stage. Either way, this is a good moment to complete another questionnaire, fill in your measurements and acknowledge how far you've come in four weeks.

It is best to come to this totally fresh and fill in the questionnaire without referring back to the one you filled out a month ago, nearer the beginning of this book. Add up your score for today, then compare it with the overall scores and those of specific areas (e.g. emotions, weight, digestive, immune, etc.), and see how you've fared. Having reached your goals, you can now learn how to transition from this point to eating healthily in everyday life in a style personalised to you. Please see page 222 for advice on reintroducing foods to your diet to find out which ones are worth including or excluding longer term to keep you healthy and to manage your weight. Your gut lining should now be in good shape, and your microbiome should be teeming with a wide range of bacteria and blooming with friendly species to provide resilience in the future. So let's get our measuring tools out again:

The Gut Makeover questionnaire

Date: _____

Rate the following symptoms on a scale of 0–5, with 0 being not present at all and 5 being a major symptom:

Emotions
Mood swings _____

Anxiety _____

Overeating _____

Feeling down _____

Trouble falling asleep, early dawn waking or sleeping too
  much _____

TOTAL _____

Weight
Bingeing (foods or drink) _____

Compulsive eating _____

Cravings _____

TOTAL _____

Digestive
Bloating _____

Acid reflux (heartburn) _____

Loose stools _____

Constipation (less than one stool movement a day) _____

TOTAL _____

Skin

Eczema _____

Psoriasis _____

Acne _____

TOTAL _____

Immune system

Hay fever _____

Asthma _____

Hives _____

Sneezing attacks _____

Stuffy nose _____

Sinus problems _____

Joint aches and pains _____

TOTAL _____

Energy

Fatigue _____

Difficulty getting up in the morning _____

Hyperactivity _____

Lethargy _____

Poor memory _____

Poor concentration _____

TOTAL _____

For women

Premenstrual symptoms _____

Menopausal symptoms _____

TOTAL _____

OVERALL TOTAL SCORE: _____

12 ways to maintain
a healthy gut

The *Gut Makeover* is a bit like a one-month makeover of a slightly shabby house where you live without paying much attention to the finer details, but then you decide to have a change. Imagine you have the builders in for a month: you get the structure improved, the cracks in the walls filled in, and the plasterers do a beautiful job finishing the walls so they are smooth. The paintwork on top is immaculate. You've had new floors put in. The doors glide open, all the screws in the handles are tightened and the squeaking hinges are silent. (This is the repair stage.) You've restored some of the existing furniture and added some new bits, too, so you have a much wider range of furniture, making best use of the space in the rooms. Then you've added the soft furnishings, beautiful rugs and cushions and plants, and you've put ornaments on the mantelpieces. (This is the reinoculation stage.)

But are you living in this house post its one-month renovation in the same way you lived in the old wreck before? Probably not.

Imagine that at the end of your house makeover you invite your friends around to celebrate. This may be done with much more ceremony than when you were living in the old version and with much more concern about red wine ending up on your new carpets!

You probably have every intention of enjoying your house to the full, but in reality you may be a bit more measured in your entertaining and spend more time on maintenance than when you lived in the old wreck. Perhaps you invest more energy in your house than before, but the enjoyment you get from living there more than makes up for the effort.

I hope that after *The Gut Makeover* you will look after your newly refurbished digestive system and enjoy the benefits in a similar way. This might involve taking more notice of what you eat and how much you drink but, with focus, the benefits (being able to better manage your weight, feeling in a better mood, having clearer skin and falling sick less often) may well outweigh the cost in terms of effort.

So, following your successful makeover, here are 12 principles for maintaining a healthy gut lining and microbiome – and all the benefits that come with it – for the long term.

1) Implement a 12-hour overnight fast habitually

After a whole month of doing this plan, you should be able to follow it literally with your eyes closed. This is a really easy practice to maintain, and can have good implications for the microbiome and consequently for metabolism and weight. Overnight, your microbiome can change – certain species come out when you are fasting and create a healthier gut lining, which in turn means less gut permeability and inflammation. An overnight fast is a convenient way of giving your gut the chance to regenerate without the inconvenience of long periods of hunger during the day, when you may be expected to perform well or don't want to risk falling into a state of hanger (hunger and anger).

2) Keep chewing, keep counting

A month of practising chewing your food properly means this may now begin to be your default eating habit. So there's no need to turn back here on this point, just keep doing what you're doing. Your gut lining and flora and consequently your overall health will be happy about this. It costs nothing, and it should make you better able to recognise when you are full so you will stop eating more than you really need to.

3) Say adios to snacks

Now that you understand the importance of including protein at each meal along with piles of fibre-rich vegetables, both of which help us to feel full up, do you really need snacks? Many *Gut Makeover* participants say their cravings for snacks are massively reduced on this plan, especially after the first week, and some found that they saved money each week by avoiding them. They also realised that when they manage the balance of each meal well, they no longer need snacks.

Often, a lot of sugar and fat comes with snacking – even healthy snacks like fruit juices and nuts – so ditching snacking is a really powerful way to keep the sugar and fat content of your diet in check and your gut lining and microbiome in good shape. High-sugar and high-fat diets can skew your gut flora and snacks can be the culprit for this. So if you remain conscious of maintaining your protein intake and fibre-rich vegetables at main meals, you shouldn't need to top yourself up with unnecessary food in between.

4) Keep up your seven a day

Forget five a day, you're now expert in seven a day! I hope that after a month on seven a day, you'll see how easy it is to eat as wide a variety as possible of vegetables, herbs and fruit as you can once you're in the swing of it.

Narrow your eyes and look at your shopping trolley as you push it towards the checkout – it should be an explosion of fresh foods teeming with bright, vibrant colours. If it looks rather more beige in tone, whip around the store again and add more colour, and more fresh food. On *The Gut Makeover* we aimed for 20–30 varieties of plants a week – one recent *Gut Makeover* participant revealed a food diary of more than 60 varieties in one week, while others were well into the 40s after a couple of weeks. And they didn't have to move to the countryside or join a remote Amazonian tribe to achieve it!

Wherever you live, try to access a wide variety of different fruits and vegetables. It's important to avoid slipping into eating beige foods and to stay focused on consuming a large range of multi-coloured foods. Your microbiome cries out for colour and variety. Feed it well.

5) Go easy on pasta and grains + choose sourdough breads

So this is where we come to the beige tone that can dominate much of the Western diet. If your gut lining and flora are in good shape, eating pasta and grains such as rice may not be a problem for you, but with the amount and domination of them in the diet they can sometimes become an issue and lead to digestive problems. We now know that the number of people who need to go gluten-free out of medical necessity is much higher than just the numbers of those who are diagnosed as coeliac, and having a resilient microbiome is key to being able to tolerate gluten. It has been observed that you are four times more likely to develop coeliac disease if you were born by C-section than if you were born vaginally. When a baby is born via the birth canal, its digestive tract is exposed (via the mouth) to bacteria from the mother's vagina. This means you start life ahead of the game with a stronger microbiome, which in turn means a stronger immune system, fewer food intolerances and less susceptibility to autoimmune disorders such as coeliac disease. After *The Gut Makeover*, your microbiome, and therefore your immune system, should be functioning better than before.

So now you may be wondering whether to go back to gluten. Later in this chapter I'll explain how you can reintroduce individual foods into your diet in stages, allowing you to observe any potential symptoms and assess if they are a real problem for you. This will give you powerful personalised dietary information to help you decide if gluten is for you or not, and to weigh up the cost versus benefit to you of having it and whether to include or exclude it long term.

The majority of people (at least 70 per cent) doing *The Gut Makeover* should be OK to go back to gluten after the month without it. If you do, here are some tips:

Choose sourdough breads such as pain Poilâne whenever you can. Sourdough breads should be easier to digest because they contain lots of friendly bacteria. Foods that are fermented are partially digested already, so can be easier on the gut.

Rotate your grains continually. Avoid a mono-grain diet. If you eat bread, choose different varieties of grain, e.g. rye or spelt. Although these both contain gluten, it is not necessarily in the same quantities as the regular dwarf wheat used in many mass-production breads. Regarding other grains, such as oats, polenta made from corn, rice and quinoa, make sure you have variety every day – it not only makes life more interesting, but it also means your gut has less chance of becoming irritated by over-exposure to one particular type of grain. In clinic, I've noticed that people who are sensitive to gluten are sometimes also sensitive to other grains. This can be rather irritating – and not just to the gut! For instance, someone goes gluten-free because of a problem with wheat, then starts consuming lots of 'gluten-free' alternatives, e.g. gluten-free beers, only to find out later that the GF beer they are drinking is made using a grain called sorghum, and they have an intolerance to sorghum, too. This is why if you have a concert of grain intolerances it may be better for your gut and health to stick to the principle of replacing grains on the plate with vegetables. Try eating a burger without a bun and instead wrapped in a couple of big lettuce leaves, or a canapé filling carried on a chicory leaf, or spiralized courgettes instead of pasta.

Go for a quality experience, rather than quantity. I recently met Dr Alessio Fasano in the coffee break of a microbiome conference in London, where he was a headline speaker. He's a leading gastroenterologist based in the United States, a pioneer of research into impaired intestinal permeability. He and his team established the first distinguishable marker of a permeable gut, a protein called zonulin. As you may have guessed from his name, he is Italian. So I asked him what kind of diet he eats, and if he eats pasta. He said he lives on a Mediterranean diet, which includes an abundance of brightly coloured plants, fish, some meat (if of good provenance), extra virgin olive oil, nuts, seeds and some red wine – which we'll come back to shortly – and one bowl of pasta a week. I liked his approach, and it makes sense.

If you don't have a known intolerance and would like to include pasta in your diet, eat a good plate of it each week and really enjoy it, but don't bombard your gut with pasta or you might risk your gut losing tolerance to it. You'll also leave more room in your diet for brightly coloured vegetables this way.

6) Invest in the least processed, most natural foods you can

I hope that after *The Gut Makeover* you'll have become a more savvy shopper and will now be used to reading the labels of all the foods you buy. Pick items with short ingredients lists and foods that sound like real foods, not food-like substances. I also hope you'll be more aware of sugar in all its different guises now, and that you will have developed a palate that demands less of it. Many *Gut Makeover* subjects report that after completing the plan they need far fewer sugary treats, such as cakes or biscuits, to get a sugar hit. If you do go for cake, go for quality over quantity – something baked with real, recognisable ingredients. If you bake yourself, you will have much more control over the amount of sugar, honey or maple syrup that you include. Do keep your radar alert for artificial sweeteners, and avoid those altogether if you can.

7) Include fermented food and drinks daily

Foods that are naturally fermented usually contain high numbers of friendly bacteria. The higher the numbers, the more chance they have of reaching the colon and doing you good. That is why I'm a fan of kefir-fermented milk, so if you can tolerate this try to include it in your diet daily somehow. You could use it as a replacement for live plain yoghurt in your foods (which probably still contains bacteria but the counts may not be as high), or desserts with fruit. If you're wondering how you know what the counts are, sadly you can't get this information easily as currently it isn't listed on labels.

Fermented pickles and sauerkraut are attracting a lot of attention among foodies and nutritionists right now. However, a lot of those sold in the supermarkets have not been slowly fermented and their labels are not clear about the length of time involved in the process or of the numbers of bacteria they contain. So if you want to obtain fermented pickles with high bacterial numbers, go to the fridge section of your health food store (the best place to find true fermented pickles these days). These should contain high numbers of bacteria; when you open the jar, it should almost burst open like a fizzy drink.

Continue to include fermented miso (bought from a refrigerated compartment) and tempeh too if you have enjoyed them on this plan. These foods have masses of friendly bacteria and can be regularly embedded in your microbiome to keep your gut healthy.

8) Use caffeine with caution

So can I go back to my beloved morning coffee, you may ask? Caffeine is a stimulant and can produce a stress response in the body, which manifests as an increase in stress hormones such as cortisol and adrenaline. When these hormones are high, our sympathetic nervous system is turned on. As explained earlier in this book, we need the other nervous system, the parasympathetic nervous system, the 'rest-and-digest' one, to be dominating when we are eating in order to digest our food well. I hope that, after a month, your rest-and-digest system has had a chance to get more into action, your digestion and absorption have improved so that food is broken down better, and dysbiosis has gone and consequently your microbiome serves you better.

So by all means enjoy caffeine, but I recommend limiting it to one really great cup of coffee daily. Coffee does contain some polyphenols, which can increase friendly bacteria, but if you have too much coffee you may risk your sympathetic nervous system becoming revved up, which means you may not digest your food so well overall and there is a danger of your digestive health suffering. Better to get your polyphenols from dark-coloured plants such as blackcurrants, blueberries, black grapes, olives, red chicory, plums, cherries, raspberries, red onions, pomegranates, or nuts and seeds such as pecan nuts or flaxseeds, or tempeh, without caffeine attached. Remember, even decaffeinated coffees and teas contain small amounts of caffeine.

9) Use extra virgin olive oil as your default oil long term

Extra virgin olive oil has been shown to make us live and look better for longer, and subjects on a Mediterranean diet with this at its base (and a wide range of vegetables and fruit) have shorter telomeres – markers of ageing. Telomeres look like strings inside our cells and shorten as we get older. However, those who use olive oil see slower shortening of these telomeres. You could call it the perfect anti-ageing food. Even when olive oil is cooked (rather than consumed raw) in the diet, the benefits to healthy ageing and a healthy heart have been shown to shine through. In the (now famous) 2013 *New England Journal of Medicine* PREDIMED study, more than 7,000 Spaniards who were at high risk of heart attack were put on a Mediterranean diet, which included 4 tablespoons of extra virgin olive oil or nuts (30g of mixed walnuts, almonds and hazelnuts) every day. The results were then compared with those of a low-fat diet group. The Mediterranean diet groups encountered up to a third less heart disease compared with the low-fat diet group, running along the same timescale (the study was halted at just under five years). The Med diet was deemed so much more effective than the low-fat one that the ethics committee cut short the study early. As for your microbiome, extra virgin olive oil contains poly-phenols, which can help the friendly bacteria flourish.

10) Get dirty

In our society there is great emphasis on good hygiene – avoid-ing dirt, vigorous hand sanitising every second that we can. It is now thought that we have become too clean, and the hygiene hypothesis suggests that not getting dirty enough is triggering a generation of atopic children. Atopic allergies are those such as eczema, asthma and hay fever. When we stroke cats, play in mud or live as part of a big family, we are exposed to lots of germs and our immune system is trained well and knows how to fight when something really dangerous comes along. However, now-adays our children often play indoors on computer screens and don't get dirty, and as a result they don't have strong immune systems to protect them from pollen, or gluten, which a robust immune system could do. A diet rich in plant diversity can help increase bacterial diversity in the gut, which primes the immune system to work well. Being less zealous with the hand sani-tiser, owning a pet, mixing with lots of people and becoming a gardener handling rotting vegetation and mud may also help.

11) Be cautious about antibiotic use

As mentioned before, antibiotics can be lifesavers, but chronic use of them for the small fry could be contributing to obesity and lowering our immune resilience. When we take antibiotics they kill the friendly bacteria in the gut as well as the pathogenic bacteria causing that ear infection, leaving us more vulnerable to getting ill again. If you do have to take antibiotics, make sure you're keeping your vegetable and fruit count at seven cups a day, that you're concentrating on lots of variety and colour, and add in kefir, Roquefort, fermented miso or tempeh for a few days, to help get the friendly bacteria in the gut flourishing again. You can do this while taking antibiotics, but it is recommended that you have these foods a couple of hours away from the time when you take your medicine, so the bacteria have a chance to embed.

12) Ring-fence a few days a week when you don't drink, especially if you are a woman

Many participants on *The Gut Makeover* said they didn't miss alcohol after a few days, and that at the end of the month they drank less in quantity, and less frequently, than they used to. They reported that cravings for alcohol reduced, and some said they felt they didn't actually need it any more to have a good time. Many found enjoyable alternatives when socialising – e.g. Virgin Mary cocktails, sparkling mineral water dressed up in a champagne flute, coconut water, or even pure watermelon juice.

It's worth remembering your gut health when and if you go back to drinking alcohol. Too much can lead to an irritated gut lining and act like weed killer on your gut bacteria, which could lower your resilience. The month spent doing *The Gut Makeover* has allowed your gut lining (which may have been irritated by chronic drinking) to heal and repopulate your microbiome.

So the big question is, how much is too much? No one knows exactly, and every one of us is different, but if you drink enough that you wake up a little dehydrated and below par the next morning, the chances are your gut may have taken a pounding, too.

There is masses of controversy around so-called 'healthy' drinking levels in the UK, and current government guidelines are no more than an educated guess at what is supposedly all right. At the moment we are being told that a 175ml glass of wine per day is 'safe' for a woman and a pint and a half of beer is safe for a man (www.drinkaware.co.uk). Doctors in the UK (principally through the Royal College of Physicians) have been pushing the government to change the current advice on talking about daily drinking quotas, and switch to weekly instead. They argue that the liver needs a rest from drinking for at least two to three days in a row each week to have time to repair itself. A healthy liver is essential for balancing our hormones and filtering out toxins so we don't develop cancer.

The microbiome has only recently been identified as an organ in its own right in the human body. I believe it is only a matter of time before drinking advice will go beyond just talking about the liver and will start to discuss protecting the microbiome, too.

Meanwhile, in 2015 a couple of hair-raising big studies added further weight to the idea that daily drinking is not a good idea. The *BMJ* paper on 136,000 people studied over 30 years showed that low to moderate alcohol intake (i.e. one glass of 175ml wine a day) increases a woman's cancer risk (predominantly breast cancer) by 13 per cent. In an accompanying editorial, one of the authors wrote: 'All people, whatever their medical history, are recommended to take a break from drinking a few days a week.' All the exact mechanisms behind the cancer link and alcohol aren't fully understood, but alcohol may lead to increased levels of the hormone oestrogen, and could be damaging DNA in our cells.

The other study weighing in on this subject was in *The Lancet*, which involved 115,000 people in 12 countries and showed that any potential benefits to heart health from wine are outweighed by the increase in the risk of cancer from alcohol consumption. The risk for cancer was 38 per cent higher in wine drinkers than those who never drank alcohol, and 20 per cent higher in beer drinkers. The bottom line is, if you're drinking wine for heart health, there is no net benefit when you add in the increased cancer risk.

Red wine contains polyphenols which – wait for it – could actually be supportive of the microbiome. Why haven't I been drinking that for the last month, you may be asking? Well, the idea behind this plan was to give your gut lining a chance to completely recover from habitual onslaught of alcohol, and to give your gut flora an uninterrupted chance to really bloom. Polyphenols are the antioxidants found in foods like extra virgin olive oil and a multitude of vegetables and fruit, as mentioned above, but you can easily and very quickly outdo any of the benefits of the polyphenols from wine with the alcohol that is also in the wine. So if you do decide to go back to wine and want to protect your microbiome and keep your cancer risk low, my advice – based on the studies above – would be the following, three times a week maximum and preferably not on consecutive days:

- Women: one 175ml glass of wine, or a G&T made with 70ml of gin, or two 125ml glasses of champagne (maximum in a single day).

- Men: a pint and a half of lager, or one 250ml glass of wine, or a large G&T, or two and a half 125ml glasses of champagne (maximum in a single day).

These numbers are way below current UK drinking guidelines (as you'll see from the drinkaware.co.uk website with its confusing unit measurements), but I think they are more in line with the latest research on cancer risks.

According to Cancer Research UK, one in two people born after 1960 will be diagnosed with cancer at some point in their life. Prevention is always better than cure, I say, and reviewing one's drinking is a good place to start.

Of course, after a month off you may decide not to go back to drinking at all. Before they started the programme, many *Gut Makeover* participants were concerned that not drinking might exclude them from social groups, but by one week into it many had already rejected this idea. They were able to see their family and friends as usual, and adapted to enjoying other drinks while socialising. One said she felt very smug waking up the next day without a hangover and bounding with energy, while her partner was a bit worse for wear.

If you are having a drink, I recommend doing so with a meal or some aperitif nibbles to cushion the impact of the alcohol on your gut lining and avoid irritation.

While on the subject of aperitifs, a tip – one small aperitif now and again could be helpful for some people's digestive systems. As I said before, we are all different, and what works for one person may not for another. But for some, particularly those who may suffer bloating after a meal, the occasional strategically positioned aperitif may actually help. This is another example of a cultural practice with a benefit and explains why traditional aperitif drinks are usually bitter concoctions by default. As I explained earlier in this book, bitter-leaf salads and lemony vinaigrettes can stimulate production of stomach acid so we break down our food better. Food that has been broken down well is less likely to cause bloating further down the digestive tract, or cause dysbiosis. Drinking a small, bitter aperitif can also stimulate production of stomach acid and lead to better digestion and less bloating in some people. The odd bitter Campari with soda water and ice, or a G&T as an aperitif washed down with a few olives (or fermented pickles), or even a nice glass of chilled dry champagne may help you out. The combination of these drinks and nibbles mean you aren't drinking on a totally empty stomach; they are also quite bitter, and if the pickles are fermented they could help your gut flora. But remember, this is beneficial in the big picture if you only drink aperitifs now and again, and not on consecutive days.

If you do end up having a few too many one evening, do some gut repair and flora help the next day. Get your chicken stock out of the freezer, heat it up with a little sea salt and sip it gently. It contains lots of electrolytes to replace those that you may have lost by drinking and the collagen helps restore your gut lining. A few sips of kefir could help, too, by planting friendly bacteria back into your microbiome.

Embracing the
Mediterranean diet

So seven plants a day, as many different varieties and colours as possible, lots of fish, some meat – particularly wild – or game, nuts and seeds, pulses (lentils, chickpeas, etc. – now your gut has repaired we can reintroduce these), sourdough bread (if you can tolerate it), extra virgin olive oil, a little red wine, a little dairy in the form of artisan-produced fermented cheeses from goats or sheep. Sounds good, doesn't it? And it could support a healthy digestive system very well, too.

That is essentially what the Mediterranean diet is, and it is easy to transition to after *The Gut Makeover*. If you follow the 12 principles in the previous chapter, your diet shouldn't be dissimilar to a real Med diet.

Some of us may not want to keep a hunter-gatherer-style diet going forever, and with just a few tweaks could benefit and enjoy a Mediterranean-style diet for the long term.

Some *Gut Makeover* participants reported that they hadn't realised how far from a natural diet their usual diet had been until they did *The Gut Makeover*, which encourages you to shine a spotlight on your usual habits. It can be surprising to discover that diet colas containing artificial sweeteners, sugary drinks and cakes, bread or pasta with most meals (meaning little rotation with other grains), highly processed tofu and soya, and processed meats containing nitrates and other preservatives and additives, all washed down with lots of caffeine, have comprised more of your original diet than you may have realised.

Post *Gut Makeover*, this is your chance to keep out the old. In the supermarket, ask yourself:

- Would I put this ingredient in this dish if I were cooking it at home?
- Would a person living in a rural village in Greece pre-1960 have eaten or drunk this?
- Would a hunter-gatherer in the Amazon easily convert to this food and remain fit, active and healthy?

A delicate gut – reintroduction of foods

One aspect of *The Gut Makeover* has involved excluding for a month certain foods known to be the most troublesome to a happy gut. These include gluten and other grains (e.g. rice, oats, couscous and quinoa), highly processed soya that has not been fermented, sugar and artificial sugars, and for omnivores, pulses (e.g. beans and lentils). In the first half of the programme, dairy from milk products was also kept at bay, and in the second half it was limited to kefir and Roquefort, which were added to the diet on a prescription basis. The diet has also been alcohol- and caffeine-free throughout. Pausing these foods and drinks not only removes potential triggers to digestive problems and potential inflammation in the gut itself, or elsewhere in the body, but also gives the digestive system a chance to recover and repair itself without the usual daily assaults it may not have been very happy about. The inside of the intestines, the villi (the shag-pile-carpet-textured area of the gut designed to provide maximum absorption for digested food), is one of the fastest-renewing areas of cells in the body. Depending on how much sensitivity to certain foods has been going on there, *The Gut Makeover* should have allowed your villi a good bit of R&R (rest and recovery) and, aided by well-digested proteins and collagen-rich stocks in your cooking, an opportunity to repair any collateral damage.

If you have suffered long-running gut issues and have felt much better over the last month, you may be feeling a little nervous about reintroducing some of the above foods. In this case I would suggest reintroducing foods in a structured manner so that you can monitor any symptoms immediately, or in the hours or days afterwards. Many medics consider the process of 'elimination and challenge' to be the gold standard for identifying food intolerances. Having done the elimination part during *The Gut Makeover* month, this may now present you with a blank canvas to do the 'challenge' detective work, to provide information for managing your health long term.

You may already have a sense of which foods might be your most troublesome from your experiences before *The Gut Makeover*. In this case, make a list of them and decide in which order you will carry out your challenges. So, decide on a food (e.g. gluten) and eat it once a day for three days and monitor your symptoms. For example, have a piece of toast or a bowl of pasta three days in a row. The reason it is better to do each challenge over three days, though it may seem like painstaking work, is that a reaction doesn't always happen immediately. Some people may bloat in the couple of hours afterwards, some not at all. Others see a worsening of a skin condition over the three days, but not immediately. There may be a return of certain immune reactions, such as coughing, asthma, watering eyes, or an itchy scalp or a very bad headache. It may be as simple as bloating, wind, or a change in stool movements (either becoming constipated or having loose stools). If you do get an instant reaction to a food, and have your answer already, there's no need to labour on with the challenge for three days. Eliminate the food from your diet and move on.

When you have the information you need, or you think everything is OK, move on to the next grain and try that. You may be OK with gluten but not with rice, for example, or OK with rice and gluten but not quinoa, and so on.

If you identify a food trigger, rejoice. You now have a potential answer to a long-running problem. If that is the case, consider removing that food from your diet for the long term, and think about how to replace the nutrients you may have received from that food from other sources. For example, the carbohydrates found in gluten and bread are also found in fruit and vegetables, so if you continue to eat seven portions of plants a day in the long term you will get plenty of carbohydrates for energy. Darker-coloured breads can be a source of B vitamins, but if you eat plenty of plants, and therefore have a healthy gut, your colon should manufacture lots of B vitamins to help the body release energy from food and also encourage good mental health. So if you replace the space on your plate with mountains of vegetables, removing gluten from your diet should not leave you in any kind of nutrient deficit.

In the second half of *The Gut Makeover*, we discussed the issue of monitoring your symptoms with the reintroduction of some milk dairy in the form of fermented milk kefir and Roquefort cheese. Fermented milk products are supposed to be easier for the digestive system to process than other types of dairy because they are already partially digested due to the fermentation process. So if you had any inkling of discomfort when you tried introducing those foods – anything from digestive symptoms to skin issues flaring up again – it may be that you have a sensitivity to either lactose or one of the proteins in milk products such as casein, and dairy is best avoided longer term if your goal is optimum health. If you do decide to remove these foods from your diet for the long term, it is even more important that you load up your plate every single day with mountains of fresh leafy green vegetables and some nuts and seeds, as many of these foods contain decent quantities of calcium needed for healthy bones, which you will need to get from elsewhere if you aren't having dairy.

Complex cases

You may have discovered a lot of new things about you and your gut on this programme, and perhaps now things are a bit better but not completely right. This may be because your gut has further underlying disturbances, causing your gut to leak and your microbiome to be out of balance (e.g. parasites, yeast infections, small intestinal bacterial overgrowth, insufficient enzymes or extensive food sensitivities – or a mixture of these). In this case I would suggest working with a nutritional therapist. Functional testing and personalised and targeted supplementation of specific strains of probiotics may be helpful.

If you are looking for a nutritional therapist in the UK, check that he or she is a member of BANT (The British Association for Applied Nutrition and Nutritional Therapy) and registered with the CNHC (Complementary and Natural Healthcare Council), which is a government-approved register. Most nutritional therapists work in the private sector. You can find one yourself by going on the BANT website: bant.org.uk/bant/jsp/practitioner-Search.faces.

Many nutritional therapists have access to, and are trained in interpreting, a wide range of cutting-edge testing from the United States and elsewhere, much of it not available on the

NHS – for example, blood tests for testing food intolerance by US-based Cyrex Laboratories and personalised genetic testing using saliva from Nordic Laboratories in Denmark. There are some comprehensive stool tests around from a range of labs, which can be invaluable if there appears to be an ongoing gut problem. These sensitive tests can pick up a wide variety of parasites and stomach bacterial infections, such as Helicobacter pylori bacteria (symptoms include nausea and chronic acid reflux), which drill holes in your stomach and can lead to stomach ulcers and cancer if left untreated. Comprehensive stool tests can measure some specific types of bacteria in the colon and give you an idea if some of the particular friendly ones are low. They also give an idea as to whether you are producing enough of the right enzymes in the gut to break down food, and if the levels of short-chain fatty acids and butyrate needed for a healthy gut lining are sufficient.

Cyrex Labs offers a blood-based, impaired intestinal perme-ability test, which measures levels of the protein marker zonulin. They also offer advanced gluten testing, but you need to be actively eating gluten for a month for an intolerance to show up on the test. If you are a complex case and need a more personal-ised approach, a well-trained, experienced nutritional therapist, who keeps in touch with your GP and/or gastroenterologist, may be the way forward.

As you'll have gathered from this book already, there is a strong link between our mind and gut. If you've ruled out all of the above issues in relation to the gut and are still having issues, it may be worth considering embarking on a talking therapy for support.

And finally, if you'd like to go DIY on the stool testing front, keep an eye on the emerging field of microbiome stool testing. The ones I've looked at so far currently don't measure the diversity and numbers of your gut flora (though that would be useful for pre- and post-*Gut Makeover*s, and this service, I am told, is coming soon). Ubiome, in the US, has just introduced a general diversity measure of gut flora comparing your levels to other subjects. Hopefully soon, Ubiome (http://ubiome.com); American Gut (http://humanfoodproject.com/americangut/) and British Gut (http://www.britishgut.org) will provide specific numbers relating to diversity of bacteria in our guts so we can measure our progress pre- and post-makeovers.

The process of change

Congratulations on finishing *The Gut Makeover*! You have made a great investment in your health, and I guarantee that your life is unlikely ever to be the same again. The knowledge you now have about the gut – your gut – will be with you for the long term. If you have reintroduced foods in a staged way, you should have been able to work out the best personalised diet for the individual you are. It may combine elements of hunter-gatherer and Mediterranean, or be more one than the other. Whether it's pulses, or dairy, processed soya, or gluten, or bolting your food, knowing the root cause of poor gut health can support good health for the long term. Once you have a picture of what works best, try to practise that style of eating long term. However, there may be setbacks and communication is going to be key.

A recent *Gut Makeover* participant, who saw her long-running gut issues disappear during the one-month plan, keeps many elements of the makeover going. She recently visited a relative whom she assumed would remember from her last visit that she is now gluten free. On arrival she was presented with a home-made lasagne, which she felt too embarrassed to not eat. She politely ate it, but told me: 'I was on the toilet, had abdominal pain and bloating for days after.' Her advice: 'Don't assume people will remember your dietary needs. You have to drop British airs and graces and be strong about communicating for the sake of your health. My relative may have taken half a day to make the lasagne but I'm sure they wouldn't have wished me a week of pain.'

Managing change

I'd like to share with you some of the thoughts that tend to go round in our minds when we make big changes in our lives. Human beings are not designed for overnight change. Change happens gradually, in stages, and I'd like to show you how far you've come in just one month.

Few people wake up one morning ready to be convinced to do *The Gut Makeover* instantly. Yes, some may, but the majority will have had to have heard the new buzz word 'gut' a few times, and to have read or heard about the links with our health and weight before coming on board. There are five stages of change and this is an example of how it may work when it comes to changing your diet:

Stage one – Denial

You hear about this book:

'I eat loads of vegetables every day. I don't need to increase them – rubbish!'

Stage two – Contemplation

You keep hearing about this book. 'Seven cups? Seven fists of plants? That sounds mad. I probably have three or four a day.'

You hear about the link between a large variety of plants each day and a healthy gut, and you hear about seven large portions being better than the standard five. You hear about the links between the gut and weight, mood, skin and immune system and start to wonder if your gut isn't as healthy as you thought – if perhaps, after all, you could ramp up your vegetable intake and widen your variety, and that there might be some major wins by doing so.

Stage three – Preparation

You buy this book. Hurray! This is the exciting bit. You're reading the book cover to cover, you're looking in your diary to identify the best four weeks to do the plan that will afford you the best chance of success.

Stage four – Action

You are actively engaging with this book. You're reducing your intake of alcohol and caffeine. You're moving on to week 1 (quite hard), week 2 (amazed at how blunted your hunger has become, and how you are enjoying the new style of eating and trying new recipes), week 3 (this is a whole new way of life!) and week 4 (I'm not sure if I want to go back to my old ways after all this). You may be actively participating on the Facebook *Gut Makeover* private group, sharing experiences, recipes and achievements and offering each other peer support.

Stage five – Maintenance

You've had success from this book and now you are looking and feeling great. In your new everyday diet you are eating seven large portions of plants a day as standard, and when you go to the supermarket you deliberately pick as many different types as possible, and continue to push the frontiers in the veg department, trying every strange new plant available. You've massively cut down on alcohol and coffee compared to before (or haven't had the urge to go back to them); when (and if) you do eat bread, it's sourdough; and you try to have a fermented food such as kefir each day. You've lost the habit of snacking, and only rarely do you crave chocolate. You might have some dark chocolate now and again in a home-made dessert or a cake, but you're more vigilant about the quality and quantities of what you put in your precious gut.

Identifying and avoiding traps

For you to sail along on the maintenance stage for the long term, do rally support from friends, family and colleagues – and perhaps even your employer. Role-modelling healthy eating often creates a better culture around you as groups tend to adopt one another's habits. You may decide to spend more time with people socially who share your health-conscious values, or have also done *The Gut Makeover*. Or you may choose to work for an employer who actively supports employees looking after their health – this might be anything from cultivating a culture of not eating at desks, providing tables or a lunch room where people can eat away from the pressures of their work, and making sure employees get proper time to rest and digest with their families when they get home, without being bombarded with emails expecting quick responses out of hours.

Be mindful. This is a four-week plan where you will learn a great deal about your gut, so you can work out the right way for you for the long term. Be aware of returning to old, unhelpful habits if they weren't working for you before. Make a commitment to the new ones that you have found really worked for you. You may even need to repeat *The Gut Makeover* from time to time for a reset, to make certain habits and food choices stick for the longer term. It's worth acknowledging that change in any of us isn't usually overnight and can involve lots of practice, time, effort and attention. Learning what combination of foods suits your gut and helps you best manage your weight varies from person to person. Once you have your best case diet established (starting with a happy gut), devote practice to it.

Also bear in mind that support from others can be very helpful to maintenance. This is why doing this plan with other people or with a friend, or having a relative taking an interest in your journey and listening and empathising, or plugging into a Facebook page regularly can help us reach and maintain our goals and make the whole experience a little more fun.

Another simple tactic to help prevent relapses is to identify your triggers. The next time you crave a bar of chocolate or make a date to meet a crowd you know will insist you binge-drink with them, try to notice what else is going on in your life at that moment. You may find there are particular emotional upsets that trigger a particular food- or drink-binge or have you phoning the heavy drinkers for a night out.

I'm going to share here my emotional food-eating trigger. It was only when I started studying nutrition and we looked at the Functional Medicine model that I was alerted to even start thinking about triggers.

Previously, if I ate an entire big packet of Kettle Chips in one sitting the voice in my head told me I was a glutton and a sloth with no self-control, and I felt a pretty nasty loathing towards myself. A bit heavy, I know, and seeing it written down here makes me think I wasn't particularly empathetic or kind to myself.

Then one day I had some upsetting news and, without even thinking about it, I stopped off at a supermarket, dashed round to the crisp section and bought a giant bag of Kettle Chips. I then walked home stuffing them down at breakneck speed until the entire contents were gone, scraping and licking the salty bits out of each corner of the bag to finish off. It might be obvious to anyone else that me being upset was my trigger for a salt binge, and I've since identified that it's the salt that gives me the kick, rather than the fat content. But I hadn't made the connection until then. Now if I'm upset, I notice the craving, and make a mental note to actively avoid Kettle Chips. I generally don't have them in the house any more for this reason. But if I am upset and feel the need for salty food, I may buy a packet of sushi instead and shake some tamari sauce on top as a healthier choice. Sushi rice, by the way, is cold and forms resistant starch, which is good for the gut, so on the maintenance part of the programme it may satisfy more than just a salt craving if you enjoy it and can tolerate rice.

Take note of what you crave next time you're upset and see if there is something that might be a better food choice instead. Or maybe it's the company of a friend who is a good listener over a cup of tea you need, rather than a night downing vodka in a big group. If you need fat and crave nuts, go for it, but an effective way to limit going overboard is to buy, or have in the house, only a 30g bag rather than the giant packs – even though they are cheaper. Even better is to remember to chew slowly. If it's chocolate, go for the darker ones with the polyphenols (another good gut nutrient – as long as it doesn't have too much sugar!). Gosh, there I go again, back to the gut . . .

Welcome to a new way of life. A healthy gut-centric kind of life.

Resources and References

For latest Gut Makeover news: www.jeannettehyde.com

Share your #gutmakeover meals on Instagram: jeannettehydenutrition

Receive #gutmakeover tips on Twitter @jeannettehyde

To check the right weight for your height, see the NHS Choices healthy weight calculator:
http://www.nhs.uk/Tools/Pages/Healthyweightcalculator.aspx

My Drink Aware – to calculate how much alcohol is in your drinks:
https://www.drinkaware.co.uk

Nutrition Data - to check the nutrient content of foods:
http://nutritiondata.self.com

To find a qualified nutritional therapist: https://bant.org.uk

To find a talking therapist: http://welldoing.org

For more information on The Institute for Functional Medicine:
https://www.functionalmedicine.org

Gut and weight

Alang, N. and Kelly, C. (2015). 'Weight gain after fecal microbiota transplantation.' *Infectious Diseases Society of America*. (2), 1.

Byrne, C., et al. (2015). 'The role of short chain fatty acids in appetite regulation and energy homeostasis.' *International Journal of Obesity*. 1–8.

Cho, I, et al. (2012). 'Antibiotics in early life alter the murine colonic microbiome and adiposity.' *Nature*. 488. (7413). 621–6.

Graham, C., Mullen, A., Whelen, K. (2015). 'Obesity and the gastrointestinal microbiota: a review of associations and mechanisms.' *Nutrition Reviews*. DOI: http://dx.doi.org/10.1093/nutrit/nuv004.

Higgins, J. (2014). 'Resistant starch and energy balance: impact on weight loss and maintenance.' *Critical Reviews in Food Science and Nutrition*. 54. 9.

Keenan, M., et al (2015). 'Role of resistant starch in improving gut health, adiposity, and insulin resistance.' *American Society for Nutrition*. 6. 198–205.

Zarrinpar, A., et al. (2014). 'Diets and feeding pattern affect the diurnal dynamics of the gut microbiome.' *Cell Metabolism*. 20. 1006–1017.

Gut and mood/brain/sleep

De Palma, G., et al. (2014). 'The microbiota-gut-brain axis in gastrointestinal disorders: stressed bugs, stressed brain or both?' *J Physiol*. 592. 14. 2989-2997.

Galland, L. (2014). 'The gut microbiome and the brain.' *J Med Food*. 17. 12. 1261-72.

Kaplan, J., et al. (2015). 'The emerging field of nutritional mental health: inflammation, the microbiome, oxidative stress, and mitochondrial function.' *Clinical Psychological Science*. 1–17.

Magnusson, R., et al. (2015). 'Relationships Between Diet-Related Changes in the Gut Microbiome and Cognitive Flexibility.' *Neuroscience*. 6.300.128-40.

Tillisch, K., et al. (2013). 'Consumption of fermented milk product with probiotic modulates brain activity.' *Gastroenterology*. 144. 7. 1394–401.

Gut and immune system

Hao, Q., et al. (2011). 'Probiotics for preventing acute upper respiratory tract infections.' *Cochrane Review*. doi: 10.1002/14651858.CD006895. pub2.

Khosravi, A., et al. (2014). Gut Microbiota Promote Hematopoiesis to Control Bacterial Infection. Cell Host & Microbe. 15. 3. 374-381.

Velasquez-Manoff, M. (2015). 'Gut microbiome. The peace-keepers.' *Nature*. 518. 11.

Gut health and autoimmune disorders (including but not limited to type 1 diabetes, Crohn's disease, ulcerative colitis, coeliac disease, multiple sclerosis, rheumatoid arthritis, psoriasis)

Campbell, A. (2014). Review article: 'Autoimmunity and the gut.' *Autoimmune Diseases*. doi.org/10.1155/2014/152428

Fasano, A. (2012). 'Leaky gut and autoimmune diseases.' *Clinic Rev Allerg Immunol*. doi: 10.1007/s12016-011-8291-x.

Matozzi, C. (2012). 'Psoriasis. New insight about pathogenesis, role of barrier organ integrity, NRL/CATERPILLER family genes and microbial flora.' *The Journal of Dermatology*. 39. 1-9.

Gut and skin conditions (rosacea, eczema, acne)

Bowie, W and Logan, A. (2011). Review: 'Acne vulgaris, probiotics and the gut-brain-skin axis – back to the future?' *Gut pathogens*. 3. 1.

Mankowska-Wierzbicka, D., et al. (2015). 'The microbiome and dermatological diseases.' *Postepy Hig Med Dosw*. 69. 978-985.

Gut and type 2 diabetes and insulin resistance

Hulston, C., et al. (2015). 'Probiotic supplementation prevents high-fat, overfeeding-induced insulin resistance in human subjects.' *British Journal of Nutrition.* 113. 596–602.

Leeman, M., Östman, E., Björck, I. (2005). 'Vinegar dressing and cold storage of potatoes lowers postprandial glycaemic and insulinaemic responses in healthy subjects.' *European Journal of Clinical Nutrition.* 59, 1266–1271.

Suez, J, et al. (2014). 'Artificial sweeteners induce glucose intolerance by altering the gut microbiota.' *Nature.* Doi10.1038/nautre13793.

Gut and autism

Mulle, J., Sharp, W., Cubells, J., (2013). 'The gut microbiome: a new frontier in autism research.' *Curr Psychiatry Rep.* 15. 2. 337.

Gut and Parkinson's

Scheperjans, F; et al. (2014). 'Gut microbiota are related to Parkinson's disease and clinical phenotype.' *Movement Disorders.* 30. 3. 350-358.

Gut and Alzheimer's

Hill, J., et al. (2014). 'Pathogenic microbes, the microbiome, and Alzheimer's disease (AD).' *Aging Neurosci.* 6. 127.

Gut, diet and cancer

Bultman, S. (2014). 'Emerging roles of the microbiome in cancer.' *Carcinogenesis.* 35. 2. 249-255.

Cao, Y., et al. (2015). 'Light to moderate intake of alcohol, drinking patterns, and risk of cancer: results from two prospective US cohort studies.' *BMJ.* doi: http://dx.doi.org/10.1136/bmj.h4238

Oyebode, O., et al. (2014). 'Fruit and vegetable consumption and all-cause, cancer and CVD mortality: analysis of Health Survey for England data.' *Journal of Epidemiol Community Health.* doi:10.1136/jech-2013-203500

Smyth, A., et al. (2015). 'Alcohol consumption and cardiovascular disease, cancer, injury, admission to hospital, and mortality: a prospective cohort study.' *The Lancet.* doi: http://dx.doi.org/10.1016/S0140-6736(15)00235-4

Gut and asthma

Huang, Y and Boushey, H. (2015). The microbiome in asthma. *J Allergy Clin Immunol.* 135. 1. 25-30.

Gut and bone health

Yang, Y., et al. (2005). 'Long-term proton pump inhibitor therapy and risk of hip fracture.' *JAMA*. 296. 24. 2947–2953.

IBS

Collins, S. (2014). 'A role for the gut microbiota in IBS.' *Nature Reviews Gastroenterology & Hepatology*. 11. 497-505.
Pozuelo, M., et al. (2015). 'Reduction of butyrate and methane-producing microorganisms in patients with irritable bowel syndrome.' *Scientific Reports*. 5. 12693.
Volta, U. (2014). 'Gluten-free diet in the management of patients with irritable bowel syndrome, fibromyalgia and lymphocytic enteritis.' *Arthritis Research & Therapy*. 16. 505.

The microbiome and dysbiosis

Beirão, et al. (2014). Review article: 'Does the change on gastrointestinal tract microbiome affect host?' *The Brazilian Journal of Infectious Diseases*. 18. (6). 660–663.
Blaser, M. (2014). 'The microbiome revolution.' *The Journal of Clinical Investigation*. 124. 10.
Clemente, J., et al. (2012). 'The impact of the gut microbiota on human health: an integrative view.' *Cell*. 148.
De Felippo, C, et al. (2010). 'Impact of diet in shaping gut microbiota revealed by a comparative study in children from Europe and rural Africa.' *PNAS*. 107. 33.
Flint, H. (2012). 'The impact of nutrition on the human microbiome.' *Nutrition Reviews*. 70. S10-S13.
Flint, H and Scott, K. (2012). 'The role of the gut microbiota in nutrition and health.' *Nature*. 9. 577–589.
Guarner, F. (2015). Review article: 'The Gut Microbiome: What do we know?' *Clinical Liver Disease*. 5. 4.
Haenen, D., Zhang, J., Souza da Silva, C., Bosch, G., van der Meer, I., Arkel, J., van den Borne, J., Gutierrez, O., Smidt, H., Kemp, B., Müller, M., Hooiveld, G. (2013). 'A diet high in resistant starch modulates microbiota composition, SCFA concentrations, and gene expression in pig intestine.' *The Journal of Nutrition*. doi: 10.3945/ jn.112.16967
Human Microbiome Project Consortium. (2012). 'Structure, function and diversity of the healthy human microbiome.' *Nature*. 486. 207–214.
Johnson, D. (2013). 'Fecal transplantation for *C difficile*: A How-To Guide.' http://www.medscape.com/viewarticle/779307
Khoruts, A. et al, (2010). 'Changes in the composition of the human fecal

microbiome after bacteriotherapy for recurrent *Clostridium difficile*-associated diarrhea.' *Journal of Clinical Gastroenterology.* 44. 354–360.

Le Chatelier, E., et al. (2013). 'Richness of human gut microbiome correlates with metabolic markers.' *Nature.* 500. 541–546.

Leach, J. (2013). Interviewed by Chris Kresser. *Revolution Health Radio Show.* 'You are what your bacteria eat: the importance of feeding your microbiome – with Jeff Leach.' November 20.

Lepage, et al. (2012). 'A metagenomic insight into our gut's microbiome.' *Gut.* DOI: 10.1136/gutjnl-2011-301805 ·

Obregon-Tito, A. (2015). 'Subsistence strategies in traditional societies distinguish gut microbiomes.' *Nature Communications.* doi:10.1038/ncomms7505

Shreiner, A., Kao, J., Young, V. (2015). 'The gut microbiome in health and in disease.' *Current Opinion in Gastroenterology.* 31 (1). 69–75.

Sun, J. (2014). Commentary. 'Artificial sweeteners are not sweet to the gut microbiome.' *Genes & Diseases.* 1. 130. 131.

Ursell, L., et al. (2012). 'The interpersonal and intrapersonal diversity of human-associated microbiota in key body sites.' *Journal of Allergy and Clinical Immunology.* 129.(5).1204–8

Van Nood, E. et al. (2013). 'Duodenal infusion of donor faeces for recurrent Clostridium difficile.' *New England Journal of Medicine.* 368. 407–415.

Van Nood, E., et al. (2014). 'Fecal microbiota transplantation facts and controversies.' *Current Opinion in Gastroenterology.* 30. 1. 34–39.

Vassallo, G., et al. (2015). Review article: 'Alcohol and gut microbiota. The possible role of gut microbiota modulation in the treatment of alcoholic liver disease.' *Ailment Pharmacol Ther.* 41 (10). 917–927.

Walker, A., et al. (2010). 'Dominant and diet-responsive groups of bacteria within the human colonic microbiota.' *The ISME Journal.* 5. 220–230.

Impaired intestinal permeability ("leaky gut")

Bischoff, et al. (2014). 'Intestinal permeability – a new target for disease prevention and therapy.' *BMC Gastroenterology.* 14.189.

Brown, K., et al. (2012). 'Diet-induced dysbiosis of the intestinal microbiota and the effects on immunity and disease.' *Nutrients.* 4. (8). 1095–1119.

Moreira, A., et al. (2012). Review article: 'Influence of a high-fat diet on gut microbiota, intestinal permeability and metabolic endotoxaemia.' *British Journal of Nutrition.* 108. 801–809.

Shen, W, et al. (2014). 'Influence of dietary fat on intestinal microbes, inflammation, barrier function and metabolic outcomes.' *Journal of Nutritional Biochemistry.* 25. 270–280.

Teixeira, T., et al. (2012). 'Potential mechanisms for the emerging link between obesity and increased intestinal permeability.' *Nutrition Research.* 32. 637–647.

The latest on cardiovascular disease and diet

Chowdhury, R., Warnakula, S., Kunutsor, S., Crowe, F., Ward, H., Johnson, L., Franco, O., Butterworth, A., Forouhi, N., Thompson, S., Khaw, K., Mozaffarian, D., Danesh, J., Angelantonio, E. (2014). 'Association of dietary, circulating, and supplement fatty acids with coronary risk: a systematic review and meta-analysis.' *Ann Intern Med*. doi:10.7326/M13-1788

De Souza, R., et al. (2015). 'Intake of saturated and trans unsaturated fatty acids and risk of all cause mortality, cardiovascular disease, and type 2 diabetes: systematic review and meta-analysis of observational studies.' *BMJ*. doi: http://dx.doi.org/10.1136/bmj.h3978

Estruch, R., et al. (PREDIMED Study Investigators). (2013). 'Primary prevention of cardiovascular disease with a Mediterranean Diet.' *The New England Journal of Medicine*. 368:1279–1290.

Harcombe, Z., et al. (2015). 'Evidence from randomized controlled trials did not support the introduction of dietary fat guidelines in 1977 and 1983: a systematic review and meta-analysis.' *BMJ Open Heart*. doi:10.1136/openhrt-2014-000196.

Malhotra, A. (2013). 'Saturated fat is not the major issue.' *BMJ*. doi: http://dx.doi.org/10.1136/bmj.f6340

Malhotra, A., DiNicolantonio, J., Capewell, S., (2015). Editorial: 'It is time to stop counting calories, and time instead to promote dietary changes that substantially and rapidly reduce cardiovascular morbidity and mortality.' *BMJ Open Heart*. doi:10.1136/openhrt-2015-000273

Smith, R. (2014). 'Are some diets mass murder?' *BMJ*. doi: http://dx.doi.org/10.1136/bmj.g7654

Coeliac disease and non-coeliac gluten sensitivity

Catassi, C., et al. (2013). Review. 'Non-celiac gluten sensitivity: the new frontier of gluten related disorders.' *Nutrients*.5. 3839-3853.

Farrell, R, and Kelly, C, (2002). Review article: 'Celiac sprue.' *The New England Journal of Medicine*. 346. 3.

Marild, K., et al. (2012). 'Pregnancy outcome and risk of celiac disease in offspring: A nationwide case-control study.' *Gastroenterology*. 142. 1. 29–45.

Rostami, K. (2012). 'A patient's journey: Non-coeliac gluten sensitivity.' *BMJ*. doi: http://dx.doi.org/10.1136/bmj.e7982.

Sapone, A., et al. (2012). 'Spectrum of gluten-related disorders: consensus on new nomenclature and classification.' *BMC Medicine*. 10. 13.

Benefits of a hunter-gatherer diet

Manheimer, E., et al. (2015). 'Paleolithic nutrition for metabolic syndrome: systematic review and meta-analysis.' *The American Journal of Clinical Nutrition.* 102. 4. 922-932.

Benefits of a Mediterranean diet

Crous-Bou, M., et al. (2014). 'Mediterranean diet and telomere length in Nurses' Health Study: population based cohort study.' *BMJ.* doi: http://dx.doi.org/10.1136/bmj.g6674

Estruch, R., et al. (PREDIMED Study Investigators). (2013). 'Primary prevention of cardiovascular disease with a Mediterranean Diet.' *The New England Journal of Medicine.* 368:1279–1290.

Petyaev, I. and Bashmakov, Y. (2012). 'Could cheese be the missing piece in the French paradox puzzle?' *Medical Hypotheses.* http://dx.doi.org/10.1016/j.mehy.2012.08.018

Simopoulos, A. (2001). 'The Mediterranean diets: what is so special about the diet of Greece? The scientific evidence.' *The Journal of Nutrition.* 131. 11.

Sofi, F., et al. (2013). Review article: 'Mediterranean diet and health.' *Biofactors.* 39. (4). 335–42.

Others

Cassidy, A., et al. (2015). 'Higher dietary anthocyanin and flavonol intakes are associated with anti-inflammatory effects in a population of US adults.' *American Journal of Clinical Nutrition.* 102. (1). 172–81.

Daskalaki, D., et al. (2009). 'Evaluation of phenolic compounds degradation in virgin olive oil during storage and heating.' *Journal of Food and Nutrition Research.* 48.1. 31–41.

Hale, L., Chichlowski, M., Trinh, C., Greer, P. (2010). 'Dietary supplementation with fresh pineapple juice decreases inflammation and colonic neoplasia in IL-10-deficient mice with colitis.' *Inflammatory Bowel Diseases.* Doi:10.1002/ibd.21320

Nobel, Y., et al. (2015). 'Metabolic and metagenomic outcomes from early-life pulsed antibiotic treatment.' *Nature Communications.* 6. 7486.

Perez-Jiminez., et al. (2010). 'Identification of the 100 richest dietary sources of polyphenols: an application of the Phenol-Explorer database.' *European Journal of Clinical Nutrition.* 64. 112–120.

Santos, C., et al. (2013). Review article: 'Effect of cooking on olive oil quality attributes.' *Food research International.* http://dx.doi.org/10.1016/j.foodres.2013.04.014

Velasco, J. and Dobarganes, C. (2002). 'Oxidative stability of virgin olive oil.' *European Journal of Lipid Science.* 104. 661–676.

Index

Acknowledgements

To all my gut clients over the past few years, thank you for teaching me so much about the digestive system and what works. Thank you to all the scientists at the coalface of this subject and informing us practitioners the other side. Thank you to all the tutors at Westminster University and the Polyclinic and in particular Heather Rosa for instilling in us your high standards.

I'm indebted to the team at Quercus and many friends and neighbours who tried out the eating plan and helped this book happen. They say it takes a village. This book certainly did. Celia and Tim, Anne, Clare, Marion and Peter, Sabine, Sarah, Imke, Rachel, Clementine, Julie, Hannah, and Fiona. Thank you for all your input. Thank you to my editor Jane Sturrock for guiding me through being a first time author and for all your enthusiasm for this subject. Thank you Jon Elek my agent for taking a punt on me.

I wouldn't have reached this point without the help of fellow nutritional therapists Marta Vazquez and Silvia Fonda – thank you for all the sharing of science papers and physiology questions together. Lisa Patient, and my BANT supervision group, thank you for all your encouragement. Thank you Ruth Hyde, my mother for role modelling healthy eating. I wish you were here to see this book. My family Markus, Hanna and Max, you've lived day-in-day-out my nine-year journey to this point. I couldn't have written this book without your love, support and encouragement.